THE **NATURAL** CANDIDA CLEANSE

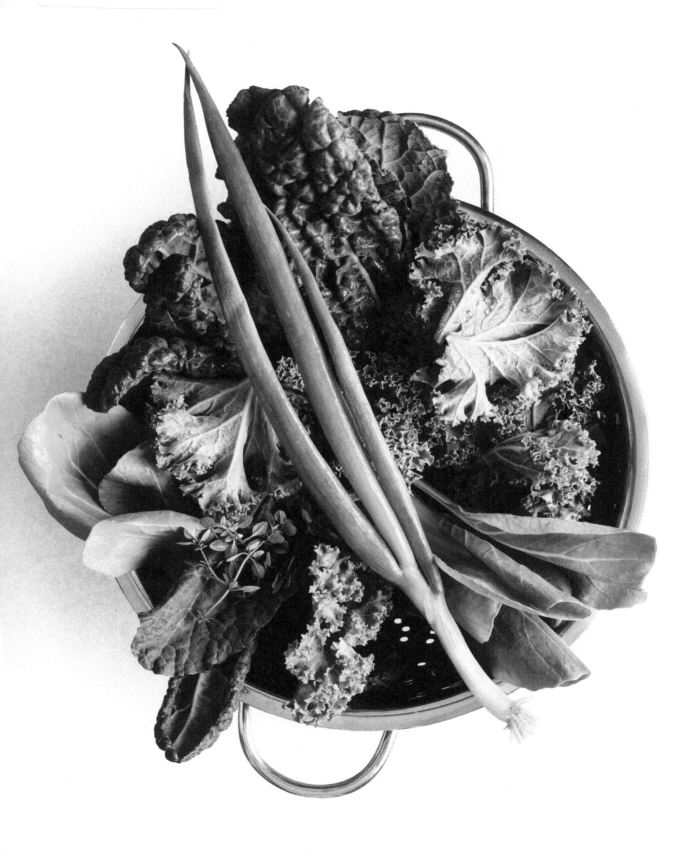

The
Natural
Candida
Cleanse

A

HEALTHY

Treatment Guide
to Improve
Your Microbiome
in Two Weeks

MOLLY DEVINE, RD

**ROCKRIDGE
PRESS**

Interior and Cover Designer: Tina Besa
Art Producer: Sue Bischofberger
Editor: Marisa A. Hines
Production Manager: Oriana Siska
Production Editor: Melissa Edeburn

Photography: © Lisovskaya/iStock, cover; © AlexRaths/iStock, cover; © Nadine Greeff, pp. ii, 95, 119, 143; © Ivan Solis, p. vi; © Fascinadora/shutterstock, p. x; © Evi Abeler, pp. 1-2, 34, 46; © Robyn Mackenzie/shutterstock, p. 20; © Victoria Wall Harris, pp. 21-22; © aaltair/shutterstock, p. 29; © Serebryakova Ekaterina/shutterstock, p. 29; © Africa Studio/shutterstock, p. 29; © Maxx-Studio/shutterstock, p. 29; © AlenKadr/shutterstock, p. 29; © Evikka/shutterstock, p. 29; © stockcreations/shutterstock, p. 35; © Pixel-Shot/shutterstock, p. 38; © MaraZe/shutterstock, p. 43; © Peiling Lee/shutterstock, p. 50; © Aaron Amat/shutterstock, p. 54; © Asya Nurullina/shutterstock, p. 66; © pr2is/iStock, p. 68; © Nataly Studio/shutterstock, p. 68; © Darren Muir, pp. 71, 110, 122, 127, 131, 138, 146; © Helene Dujardin, pp. 74, 100, 105, 115, 124; © Marija Vidal, p. 77; © Linda Schneider, p. 80; © Dani Vincek/shutterstock, p. 85; © MaraZe/shutterstock, p. 140.

ISBN: Print 978-1-64152-660-9 | eBook 978-1-64152-661-6

R1

For Brent, Harper, Luke, Evan, Geege, and Dats. I couldn't ask for better companions in the love of food, health, and happiness.

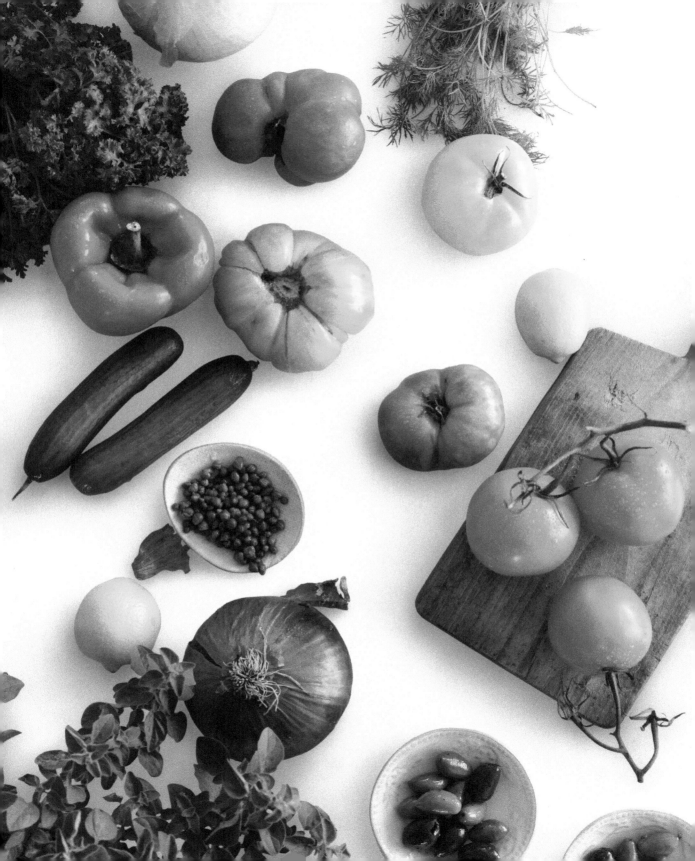

CONTENTS

INTRODUCTION

I was diagnosed with Hashimoto's thyroiditis, an autoimmune hypothyroid condition, when I was 12 years old. I swam competitively and, even as a preteen, was practicing twice a day most days. I did not have any of the clinical symptoms of hypothyroidism, which I attribute to my young age and very active lifestyle. My diagnosis was made when my pediatrician discovered an enlarged gland during a routine physical. I was well managed on synthetic thyroid hormone therapy through puberty, college, adulthood, and three pregnancies. Throughout it all, I never gave my thyroid or autoimmune condition a second thought—until it reminded me it was there and started manifesting itself in unpleasant ways.

In my midthirties, I started to experience gut issues that ranged from extreme bloating, gas, and diarrhea to nausea and constipation: in other words, textbook irritable bowel syndrome (IBS). When my 12-year-old daughter casually mentioned after school one day that her friend had asked if I was pregnant again, I knew I could not live like this forever. As a registered dietitian, I was determined to get to the bottom of this often-embarrassing digestive discomfort and settled upon a process of elimination diet and supplementation. I tried low FODMAP (avoiding all short-chain carbohydrates: Fermentable Oligosaccharides, Disaccharides, Monosaccharides, and Polyols), dairy-free, gluten-free, and low glycemic index, but found little relief. I took digestive enzymes, L-glutamine, and collagen (all of which I discuss in chapter 3; see "What Happens in This Process?," page 51), which helped some, and yet I rarely could eat a meal without immediately watching my stomach blow up like a balloon. Also, because I was a former personal chef and lover of all things food, being so restrictive with my meals without experiencing total relief was incredibly frustrating to me.

It was not until I tried the ketogenic approach for a few weeks while working on a recipe project for a supplement company that I found complete digestive relief. I went from not being able to eat a thing without immediate discomfort and bloating to enjoying meals with friends and family without feeling inclined to wear maternity clothes to every event! This was primarily because a ketogenic diet derives most of its nutrition (or calories) from fat sources, while being moderate in protein and very low in carbohydrates. It excludes all sugars, refined carbohydrates, low-fat dairy, most fruits, grains, legumes, and starchy vegetables. Despite being fairly restrictive of carbohydrates, my diet gave me such relief that I was extremely motivated to continue it and to share my experience with my clients.

There are striking similarities between a ketogenic approach and an elimination diet for candida overgrowth, as well as the diseases and conditions each help improve. I began to employ the principles I had learned from my personal experience to help my clients overcome their symptoms of IBS, food intolerance, inflammation, joint pain, stubborn weight gain, and many others. I was able to do so successfully, without leaving them feeling hungry or deprived or bored with their food choices. As I suspected, so many of their conditions were merely *symptoms* of a greater underlying root cause: candida overgrowth, or *candidiasis*. Once we addressed the root cause of disease, the symptoms of that disease simply went away. I was able to help my clients find a sustainable, long-term approach to keep their candida under control, which eliminated their symptoms and allowed them to enjoy some of their favorite foods in moderation.

I am a registered and licensed dietitian by training, holding a certificate of training in integrative and functional nutrition from the Academy of Nutrition and Dietetics. I have undergone rigorous training, including the completion of 1,200 hours of supervised practice through a dietetic internship program accredited by the Accreditation Council for Education in Nutrition and Dietetics, and I passed the Commission on Dietetic Registration's registration examination for credentialing. Because of what I learned in my formal training, I do not subscribe to "fad diets" or nutrition "magic bullets." I believe food is medicine and is the key ingredient to overall health, but we must not ignore other lifestyle factors. I believe in treating the whole person. In chapter 3, when I discuss the heart of the treatment plan, I will touch on the four pillars of health: nutrition, emotional well-being/stress, sleep, and physical activity. All play a vital role in disease prevention and in achieving optimum health.

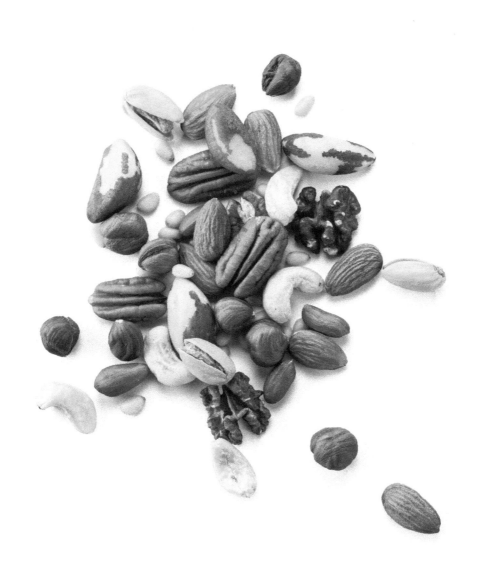

PART I

Living with Candida Overgrowth

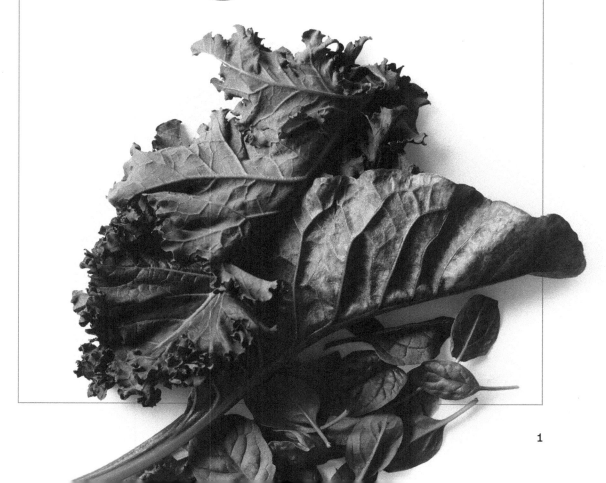

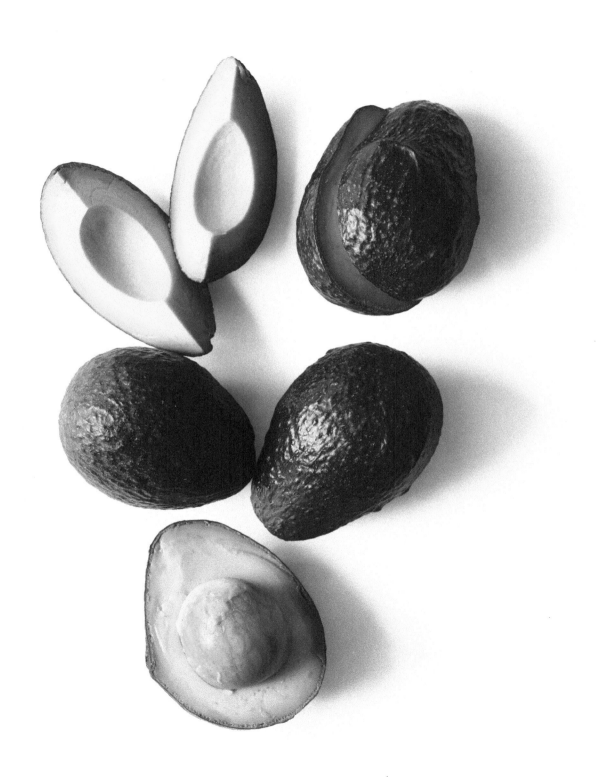

CHAPTER ONE

Understanding
Candida

*C*andida is a form of yeast colonizing the microbiota of most humans and mammals. When kept in balance with other microorganisms such as bacteria, it is harmless and causes no adverse symptoms. However, when this balance gets disturbed through poor diet, antibiotic use, hormone replacement, chronic stress, and other environmental toxins, the candida yeast spreads as a fungus to form candidiasis infection. Research suggests that candida infection may be to blame for many diseases of the gastrointestinal (GI) tract such as Crohn's, ulcerative colitis, and gastric ulcers.

The first reported description of candida infection was in 1839 by German scientist Bernhard von Langenbeck.[1] Since that time, candidiasis has been primarily studied and accepted as either oral thrush (oropharyngeal candidiasis) or vaginal yeast infection (vulvovaginal candidiasis).[2] Due to a lack of definitive testing measures and a still very young study of the gut microbiome, GI candidiasis is a relatively understudied and under-accepted condition that is affecting an ever-increasing population. As a result of this gap in knowledge among most healthcare professionals, many cases of GI candidiasis are going undiagnosed and causing a host of other treatable inflammatory conditions, including food intolerance and inflammatory bowel conditions. While I do not believe that candidiasis is at the root of *every* inflammatory or autoimmune condition under the sun, I do strongly support the implementation of an anti-candida dietary approach to attack the root cause of many digestive, skin, and inflammatory conditions.

Understanding Candida Overgrowth

While over 150 different species of *Candida* exist, *Candida albicans* is the most prevalent in humans and the most common culprit of infection. In its benign state, *Candida albicans* is a harmless member of a balanced and healthy human microbiome. Present in more than 70 percent of the population from the time of birth, it colonizes the oral cavity, gastrointestinal tract, and genitourinary (urinary and reproductive organ) tract. Unfortunately, in our modern world of poor diet, high stress, poor sleep, environmental toxins, and overuse of antibiotics and birth control, the gut microbiome can become very imbalanced, allowing the once benign *Candida albicans* to spread beyond the GI tract. In a healthy microbiome, the epithelial cells that line the GI tract have tight junctions and don't allow toxins or bacteria to leave the gut. However, when these cells become compromised, the barrier they create also becomes compromised, allowing bad bacteria and infection to enter the bloodstream, causing systemic inflammation that can lead to many life-threatening infections.

A healthy gut microbiome consists of about 80 percent "good" microorganisms to about 20 percent bad bacteria, yeast, and fungi. With the regular consumption of probiotics, limited sugar and refined carbohydrate intake, and minimal antibiotic or immunosuppressive therapy drug use, the 20 percent is natural and kept under control, allowing healthy GI function to persist.

If our gut microbiome naturally wants to live in harmony, why is gut dysbiosis and its associated complications becoming more prevalent? The answer lies in our day-to-day habits that have become such a part of fast-paced modern life that we often overlook the negative impact they can have on our health. Researchers have theorized that there are four main culprit areas:

Most Americans eat a poor diet. Americans are consuming more sugar and processed foods than ever before. The average American consumes 66 pounds of added sugar each year. Combine that with the gut-disrupting chemicals and additives in processed foods and a lack of micronutrients from fresh vegetables, and the gut microflora loses its integrity.

We are killing off the good bacteria. Antibiotics are consistently overprescribed, even when patients are very young. As a result, antibiotic-resistant strains of bacteria develop, and the loss of the good bacteria to defend against other pathogens creates a compromised immune system, perpetuating the vicious cycle.

Birth control is being started at earlier ages in young girls. Studies have shown a correlation between the prevalence of candidiasis and the use of oral contraceptives and hormone replacement therapy (HRT) containing estradiol. This is primarily due to an increase in glycogen (the stored form of glucose) in the epithelial cells, which subsequently provides a steady food source for the fungal infection.

We are overstressed and sleep deprived, resulting in chronically elevated cortisol levels. While acute levels of stress and cortisol (the body's main stress hormone) help protect us from danger and increase our immune system, chronically elevated levels lead to a suppression of immunity, leaving us vulnerable to infection and disease.

All of these factors together create a perfect recipe for disaster. As we kill off our protective gut bacteria with antibiotics and weaken our immune systems with chronic stress, poor sleep, and immunosuppressive agents such as corticosteroids to treat asthma, arthritis, and allergic reactions, we create an environment ripe for the overgrowth of yeast and fungi.[3] This overgrowth is then accelerated by the introduction of excessive amounts of refined sugars and processed foods in the standard American diet, thus allowing the growing *Candida* to take advantage of a compromised immune system.

In addition to the top four theorized connections, we are also beginning to learn more about the relationship between diabetes mellitus (DM) and candidiasis. *Candida* can provoke an elevated level of insulin secretion, which increases the chances for the onset of DM. Similarly, patients with chronically elevated blood sugar, or uncontrolled diabetes, have higher rates of candidiasis in the form of frequent yeast infections and oral thrush because their uncontrolled disease allows for a steady food source for the growing infection (glucose) as well as a compromised immune system that can't fight off the spread of infection. As with many conditions, it begs the age-old question about the chicken or the egg. In some cases, DM may have been brought on by the *Candida* and its demands for insulin, thus causing stress on the pancreas, resulting in insulin resistance and decreased insulin output. In other cases, the disease created a perfect environment for *Candida* overgrowth that previously did not exist. We may never know which came first in many cases, but the treatment for candidiasis and DM is clear: Decrease glucose and starve off the *Candida*.

If you have ever baked bread, you know the first step is to activate the dormant dry yeast. To do so requires a warm environment (of which the human body temperature of 98.6 degrees Farenheit would certainly qualify), liquid (of which the human body has plenty), and something for yeast to feast upon (honey or sugar are favorites for quick activation). Within a few minutes, the yeast begins to awaken, create gas bubbles, and GROW. The same thing happens inside your GI tract when the candida yeast is given a steady source of food and has a diminished population of defending microorganisms to stop it. It is a recipe for digestive discomfort, inflammation, food intolerances, skin reactions, and endocrine disruption. As the candida infection grows, it is able to penetrate the epithelial cells of the stomach and small intestine, eventually spreading into the bloodstream, causing systemic inflammation. I believe that most food intolerances and diagnoses of IBS, as well as many cases of chronic joint pain and skin irritations, are actually *symptoms* of candidiasis and can be mitigated by treating the root cause: candida overgrowth.

Through both my personal and professional experience battling and overcoming candidiasis, I have learned that the cause of infection can often be multifaceted. I do believe that in today's world, it is hard to avoid an onslaught of potential triggers. For me, underlying autoimmunity likely caused a hotbed of opportunity for infection and overgrowth. Recurring urinary tract infections, sinus infections, and a bout of mononucleosis were all signs of reduced immunity and potential opportunity for infection. Frequent doses of antibiotics to treat these conditions only led to a further compromised gut microbiome and decreased immunity. If I could go back in time and apply what I know now, I would have saved myself a decade of GI discomfort, frustration, and food elimination. I want to share my knowledge and expertise with you to stop candidiasis in its tracks once and for all so you can resume happy and healthy living!

Symptoms

Candida albicans is the most common human pathogen and causes a multitude of symptoms ranging from superficial skin and mucosal to life-threatening systemic inflammation and infection.[4] Some individuals only exhibit one or two symptoms whereas others find that they can relate to most of the symptoms described in the following paragraphs. Typically, the more invasive the candidiasis and the longer the duration of infection, the more widespread and systemic symptoms can be.

Digestive complications: These are typically the most common symptoms that bring clients to my office seeking relief. Digestive symptoms range from simple discomfort (bloating, gas, diarrhea, constipation, and intense sugar cravings) to life-impacting sudden food intolerance and intense abdominal pain. As the Candida grows and spreads, it requires more and more food to continue flourishing in the GI tract. This causes the host to crave sweets, refined carbs, breads, pastas, and rice, which then only fuel the fire of overgrowth. As the Candida grows, it releases carbon dioxide gas, which causes the host to have excessive abdominal bloating, belching, and flatulence. The complications from Candida overgrowth often occur after meals, although they can be constant throughout the day in some cases, leading the host to assume they have developed a sudden food intolerance or allergy. Then, the cycle of food elimination comes into play but rarely brings relief because the food

Common Misperceptions about Candida

Today, we have immediate access to more information than ever before. In the landscape of health and wellness, this wealth of information has its pros and cons. While so much information can be a helpful and convenient resource, information overload is a constant source of struggle for many of my clients. Conflicting advice and opinions (usually not rooted in scientific evidence) lead to confusion, inflated and often unfounded expectations for a magic-bullet cure, and ultimately frustration with protocols that just don't live up to their hype. A functional and integrative approach to health looks at addressing the root cause of illness rather than treating its symptoms alone. We must take a step back and look at the many pieces that make up each individual human puzzle to determine a sustainable and effective treatment plan.

The Natural Candida Cleanse is designed to attack the root cause of the host of symptoms associated with candida overgrowth. Keeping the whole person in mind, including all lifestyle factors, we can debunk some common misconceptions about *Candida* and its treatment.

Claim 1

You need an extreme cleanse to effectively starve off infectious *Candida*.

FALSE! We don't need to starve our bodies of essential micro- and macro-nutrients—only those that specifically cause the yeast to thrive. In fact, malnutrition can cause other stress on our bodies, which only worsens the condition.

Claim 2

Ridding your body of harmful candida fungus will cure all conditions and alleviate all symptoms.

FALSE! Yes, a happy and healthy gut is vital to a happy and healthy life, including immune function, digestion, healthy weight maintenance, reduced inflammation, and risk for chronic disease, just to name a few aspects. However, it is important to remember that the human puzzle has many pieces. As a dietitian, I believe food is our best medicine. I also respect that certain conditions arise out of factors unrelated to diet and lifestyle and must be treated accordingly.

Claim 3

Addressing nutrition alone will eliminate all symptoms associated with candida overgrowth.

FALSE! We are more than the sum of our parts. Lifestyle factors outside of nutrition such as a toxic environment, poor sleep, and high stress can cause oxidative damage to our cells, which can result in symptoms that mimic those of candida overgrowth.

Claim 4

The goal of the Natural Candida Cleanse is to rid the body of ALL candida.

FALSE! Candida is the most common fungus in the human body, and while some species can cause infection, not all species are harmful. In fact, we need both good AND bad fungus and bacteria to sustain symbiosis and healthy gut function.

Claim 5

Killing off infectious candida alone will lead to long-term success.

FALSE! While it is important to starve the harmful candida organisms to cause "die-off," we must introduce good bacteria in the form of probiotics and fermented foods to sustain balance and prevent future gut dysbiosis.

is not the root cause of the discomfort; rather, the *Candida* causes the chain reaction. Many of my clients have come to me assuming they have a dairy, gluten, or soy intolerance due to their IBS symptoms when, in reality, the sugar in these dairy-, wheat-, or soy-containing foods was fueling their discomfort.

Physical complications: While digestive symptoms may be the uncomfortable complications that prompt my clients to seek relief, I often see many associated physical symptoms in those with *Candida* overgrowth. Most common are weight gain despite efforts to maintain a healthy weight, skin irritations, joint pain, fatigue, and nail fungus, vaginal yeast infection, and oral thrush. Oropharyngeal candidiasis (oral thrush) and vulvovaginal candidiasis (vaginal yeast infection) are the most clinically accepted forms of *Candida* yeast infection in traditional medicine, but I find that only a handful of my candida clients exhibit these symptoms. More common and less obvious in those with GI candidiasis are weight gain and joint pain. Both of these are a result of the systemic inflammation caused by the candidiasis, as well as the change in dietary habits that result from intense sugar cravings and consumption to keep their candida population happy and thriving. Due to chronically elevated blood glucose levels, increased insulin secretion, and weight gain, these individuals are at a higher risk for developing type 2 diabetes mellitus.

Cognitive and psychological complications: As we begin to better understand the important gut-brain connection, we are learning more and more about the impacts of poor digestive health on cognitive function, as well as on cognitive decline. Also known as the enteric nervous system, our gut is sometimes referred to by scientists as our second brain because they are finding more and more evidence that irritation and infection in the GI system may send signals to the central nervous system (CNS) that trigger mood changes.[5] Researchers at Johns Hopkins University found that a history of *Candida* yeast infections was more common in individuals with schizophrenia or bipolar disorder,[6] and it is believed that exposure to infectious organisms during critical stages of neurodevelopment may cause damage to the CNS, resulting in the onset of behavioral anomalies and psychiatric disorders during adulthood.[7] While further research is needed to determine a cause-and-effect relationship between candida overgrowth and mental health, it is clear that the two are associated. Common psychological symptoms in individuals suffering from candidiasis include brain fog, poor memory, depression, anxiety, and food addictions. Not only does the systemic infection and resulting inflammation have a negative impact on brain health, but glucose overload and insulin spikes triggered by increased sugar and starch consumption in response to cravings also negatively impact the mitochondria of the brain and may lead to a greater risk for neurological conditions such as Alzheimer's and dementia.

What Is Leaky Gut Syndrome?

It is very common for individuals with candida overgrowth to also have *leaky gut syndrome*, or intestinal permeability. Leaky gut occurs when there is a breakdown of the epithelial lining of the stomach and intestine, causing gaps or holes in this vital protective barrier. We know that leaky gut plays a role in certain GI conditions such as celiac disease, Crohn's disease, and IBS, and there is growing evidence that the standard American diet and other stressors of modern-day life contribute to this condition. Poor diet, stress, heavy alcohol use, and frequent use of anti-inflamatory drugs (NSAIDs) can all cause deterioration of the intestinal barrier, allowing toxins, antigens, and bacteria to enter the bloodstream and initiate widespread inflammation, bowel irregularity and discomfort, and increased risk for infection. Growing evidence shows that in individuals with a genetic predisposition, a leaky gut may allow environmental toxins to enter the body and trigger the development of autoimmune disease. A healthy gut microbiome is important in maintaining epithelial lining integrity and is imperative for restricting environmental toxins from entering the bloodstream. Candidalysin, a pore-forming peptide toxin that is secreted by invading infectious *Candida albicans*, was recently discovered to be a crucial determinant in epithelial cell damage. Another chicken-or-egg conundrum: Does candida infection cause leaky gut or does a preexisting leaky gut brought on by environmental toxins and a poor diet allow for the invasion of *Candida* and resulting gut dysbiosis? Both are likely to blame to some degree, but regardless, candidiasis and leaky gut often go hand in hand.

When to Talk with Your Practitioner

While the candida cleanse through dietary intervention, or Natural Candida Cleanse, outlined in chapters 2 and 3, is designed to rid your body of harmful candida overgrowth, in some cases, intervention through a trained and experienced healthcare professional may be necessary. As a functional and integrative nutrition practitioner, I believe that food is medicine. However, one of the tenets of integrative medicine is that its therapies often are used in combination with traditional medical intervention for a comprehensive approach to certain conditions.

If your symptoms are primarily digestive (e.g., bloating, gas), cognitive (e.g., mental fog, lack of concentration), or psychological (e.g., depression, anxiety) without any physical manifestations of candida infection, a registered dietitian specializing in integrative nutrition or an integrative clinician will be able to assess your symptoms and order tests to properly diagnose and treat your condition.

For individuals with extensive candidiasis manifesting itself on the skin in ways such as oral thrush, vaginal yeast infection, nail fungus, or other skin irritations, the use of topical or oral antifungal agents in combination with dietary intervention may be necessary to completely eradicate the infection. If you suffer from persistent vaginal yeast infections, or nail infections or display symptoms of oral thrush (such as white spots in your mouth that resemble cottage cheese, redness at the corners of your mouth, a painful sensation in the mouth, or difficulty swallowing), it may be time to make an appointment with your primary care provider.

PREPARING FOR YOUR VISIT: WHAT TO EXPECT

A registered dietitian or integrative clinician will focus on physical symptoms, medical history, medications, recent lab values, and dietary and lifestyle habits. A trained and experienced provider can often deduce a diagnosis of probable candidiasis from this information alone. In more complicated cases, additional tests may be appropriate or necessary.

Testing options include:

Blood test: Looks for high levels of immunoglobulins, which are antibodies in the blood that are indicative of a candida infection.*

Comprehensive stool analysis (CSA): Cultures for bacteria and yeast in the stool as well as inflammatory markers indicating infection. Two stool samples must be collected on two separate days and received in the lab within seven days of the first testing day.

Urine test: This tests for the presence of a waste product of pathogenic or infectious *Candida* called D-aribinitol in the urine. A positive result is indicative of candidiasis.

Stool and urine tests can be ordered by both registered dietitians and integrative clinicians through third-party testing services. Registered dietitians cannot order blood tests, but they can work with your primary care provider to request these. Results typically take a couple of weeks but may take up to a month. While many nutrition counseling appointments with registered dietitians are covered by insurance, testing is typically an out-of-pocket expense. Although most testing is not covered by insurance, some testing that is carried out through integrative medical clinics may be covered under some plans. Out-of-pocket costs typically range from $100 to $400.

HOW THE MEDICAL FIELD VIEWS CANDIDA

Many traditional medicine practitioners have little background knowledge or a full understanding of the gut microbiome and its important role in disease prevention and overall health. For that reason, it is best to seek out a nutrition professional or integrative practitioner who has more experience

---

* Of note: In September 2014, the FDA gave marketing approval for the T2Candida Panel, the first direct blood test for detecting five Candida species that cause bloodstream infections. This is a rapid blood test that produces results in three to five hours but is found only in large medical facilities such as hospitals or large outpatient clinics.

with a holistic, whole-body approach to medicine. While oropharyngeal candidiasis (oral thrush) and vulvovaginal candidiasis (vaginal yeast infections) are widely accepted in the traditional medical community, mainly because they can be observed, easily diagnosed, and treated with antifungal medications, the concept of candidiasis of the gastrointestinal tract without other physical symptoms is often eschewed. Those of us who specialize in digestive disorders and food intolerance, however, have a deep understanding of the complex relationship between a balanced microbiome and overall health and sustained well-being.

Even in the community of medical providers who promote healthy gut function as an integral component of disease prevention, there is limited research on the role fungi play on gut homeostasis, and there is a lot of education to be done regarding *Candida*, gut dysbiosis, and systemic inflammation. We know that dietary intervention is imperative to restore gut balance and rid the body of candida infection, but there are also antifungal medications and over-the-counter (OTC) supplements that may be prescribed in conjunction with dietary intervention.

WHAT IS NORMALLY PRESCRIBED?

Most common topical and oral antifungal medications and generic names

For cutaneous candidiasis (infections occurring externally on the skin), topical antifungal creams are often prescribed. Most common are Nystatin, clotrimazole, econazole, ciclopirox, and miconazole. For persistent infection, vulvovaginal candidiasis, oropharyngeal candidiasis, or cutaneous candidiasis that does not respond to topical treatment, oral medications such as fluconazole or itraconazole are prescribed with therapies ranging from three to six months and often must be repeated for several cycles.[8]

How oral medications might interact with common drugs and prescriptions

While these oral therapies can help kill off infection in many, they may not be long-term solutions without proper lifestyle change and dietary intervention. Additionally, these therapies come with potential side effects and drug interactions that may cause more harm than benefit. These risks can be easily avoided through other intervention modalities.

Side effects of the commonly prescribed fluconazole include headache, dizziness, drowsiness, stomach or abdominal pain, diarrhea, heartburn, allergic reactions including rash or itching, and unpleasant taste. As these are also often symptoms associated with candidiasis, you may not recognize if you are having a negative reaction and may realize you are finding relief from a therapy combined with diet intervention.

Fluconazole may interact negatively with certain antibiotics, blood thinners, diuretics, sedatives, antiseizure drugs, and certain other medications.

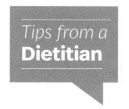

Tips from a **Dietitian**

Many of my clients have suffered for years from digestive discomfort and the associated symptoms that come with it. Bloating, bowel changes, stubborn weight gain, fatigue, depression, brain fog, and joint pain are just a few of the many symptoms that lead clients to my door. Most of these infirm individuals have sought out a dietitian because they believe a food allergy or intolerance is to blame or that simply by following a reduced-calorie meal plan, they will finally see improvement in the way they feel. For many, their primary care provider has told them they "need to lose weight" or "exercise more," placing blame on the patient. They feel defeated, inadequate, and immensely frustrated with their health. It has never occurred to them that there may be a deeper root cause of their host of symptoms and that they may be a victim of infection rather than the culprit of their own poor health.

If you are reading this book, you understand that an overgrowth of *Candida albicans* may be to blame for the symptoms you are experiencing, and you are ready to defeat it! Remember that healing takes time and effort, but it does not have to feel like an uphill battle. Our bodies are incredibly resilient, and we have so many protective mechanisms in place already if we give those systems the ability to do their jobs. It is important to trust your body's natural ability to heal. During the next few weeks, therapeutic nutrition is your job. If you give your body the proper fuel, it will be able to do its job and restore balance to resume healthy function.

Holistic Healing at Home

WHEN IS IT TIME/SAFE TO TAKE MATTERS INTO YOUR OWN HANDS?

I will say it again: Food is medicine! The therapeutic dietary protocol outlined in chapters 2 and 3 is your prescription for better health. If your symptoms are primarily digestive, cognitive, or psychological, it is likely that a dietary intervention will improve these symptoms without need for medication or a visit to your practitioner. Remember, *Candida albicans* is a perfectly normal member of the human gut microbiome and likely has been in your system since birth. The environmental factors of modern life (primarily poor diet, stress, and prescription medication use) allowed it to grow out of control and become infectious. Candida thrives on glucose from sugars and many carbohydrates and needs this fuel to survive. By depriving it of its main source of energy for life, you can kill off the large invasive population of candida infection, replenish your natural protective gut bacteria, and regain your health. Through holistic lifestyle change, we have the ability to heal our bodies from the inside out.

While I believe that dietary intervention alone can kill off the invading infection and restore balance and health in many individuals, some infections may be more widespread and require additional intervention. If symptoms do not improve within two to four weeks (not all will be fully resolved, but there should be a noticeable improvement), it may be time to consult a trusted medical provider.

Additionally, individuals experiencing the following symptoms should consult a physician prior to starting any nutrition therapy, as these may need more immediate attention:

- → Blood in stool or urine
- → Vomiting
- → Severe abdominal pain that is constant
- → Swelling in legs
- → Lightheadedness or feeling faint
- → Blurred vision
- → Tingling sensation in extremities
- → Severe thirst or frequent urination
- → Chest pain
- → Shortness of breath or trouble breathing

Individuals who are severely immunocompromised, such as those with HIV or AIDS, undergoing cancer treatment, or with uncontrolled diabetes, should consult their primary care provider because medication intervention is likely also required.

Individuals on insulin therapy should consult their primary care provider before beginning any dietary protocol because dosing may need to be adjusted to compensate for lower carbohydrate intake.

REASONS TO TAKE A HOLISTIC APPROACH AS OPPOSED TO MEDICATION

We are a population that is overmedicated and undernourished. Too often, we look for an "easy button," often in the form of a pill or medication. Traditional medicine has a long history of mitigating symptoms without addressing the root causes of illness. The number of prescription medications individuals are taking mounts while health does not improve, and ironically, many of these medications negatively interact with one another or cause other side effects requiring additional medication. It is a vicious cycle. If traditional medicine practitioners took the time to educate their patients about the influence of nutrition, sleep, stress, and physical activity on health, they would be able to reduce the number of prescriptions written and provide their patients with a long-term solution for overall health and disease prevention.

By following the dietary protocol outlined in chapters 2 and 3, you will not only be able to heal your body from the inside out without prescription medication or traditional medicine intervention but you will also learn valuable tools to incorporate sustained lifestyle changes that promote long-term health and disease prevention. Holistic healing is not a Band-Aid for a symptom; rather, it is a cure for the problem.

CASE STUDY

Lisa came to me looking for relief from her symptoms of self-described "IBS." Despite being a very slender woman in her late fifties (and postmenopausal), she was frustrated by her "pregnant belly" every time she ate. She attributed this excessive bloating and digestive discomfort to some sort of food intolerance or allergy and was looking for nutrition counseling and dietary intervention to get to the bottom of it. She had eliminated dairy from her diet, as she was sure this was the culprit of her discomfort, but the bloating persisted.

As I began to examine her medical history and other symptoms, I came to learn Lisa also was suffering from recurrent fungal nail infections despite the use of topical antifungal creams, trouble swallowing and a feeling of airway restriction after meals (which she also attributed to food intolerance), and lifelong asthma for which she had been using inhaled steroid therapy via a nebulizer almost daily for several years. The previous year, she had developed pneumonia from a stubborn upper respiratory infection and was put on two rounds of prednisone to treat it. She complained of fatigue and irritability and reported that she just felt "off." While Lisa ate a fairly healthy diet by most standards, she was consuming a large amount of processed and refined carbohydrates in the form of crackers, bread products, and cereals. In an effort to eat more healthily, she had also included many fruits and whole grains such as quinoa and brown rice into her diet. Her animal protein intake was low and she avoided high-fat foods. From a quick analysis, I determined she was easily consuming approximately 75 to 80 percent of her daily calories from carbohydrate sources alone.

Without performing any diagnostic testing, I went on the hunch she had a classic case of candidiasis that was presenting itself physically as well as psychologically. Her history of corticosteroid use for infection as well as asthma left her immune system fragile and microbiome unbalanced. *Candida* had an opportunity to multiply when her self-prescribed elimination diet left her eating high levels of starchy foods, and the overgrowth then presented itself physically on her hands and in her throat. I quickly put her on my Natural Candida Cleanse protocol, recommended an OTC probiotic, and included probiotic foods such as kefir, kimchi, and small amounts of yogurt to restore gut health. At our first two-week follow-up appointment, she reported drastically improved digestion and was thrilled to tell me she was able to go to business lunches now without fear of embarrassment from excessive bloating. After having previously restricted so many foods she believed were the source of her problems and/or "unhealthy," she now considered her diet to be the most varied it had been in over a year. Her nail fungus persisted, but as she continued with antifungal creams, this too cleared up after the first month. Her asthma was also better managed with only occasional need for the nebulizer.

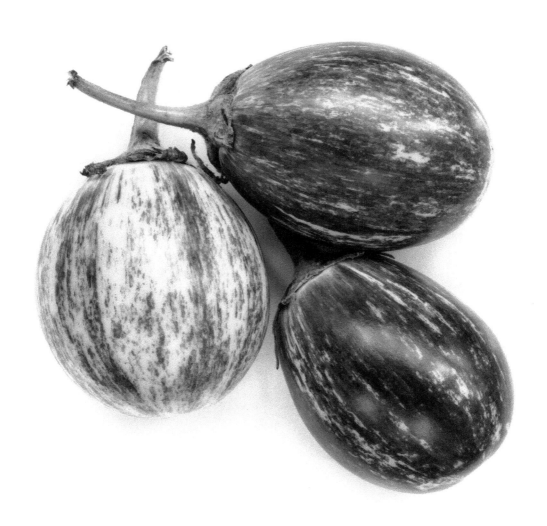

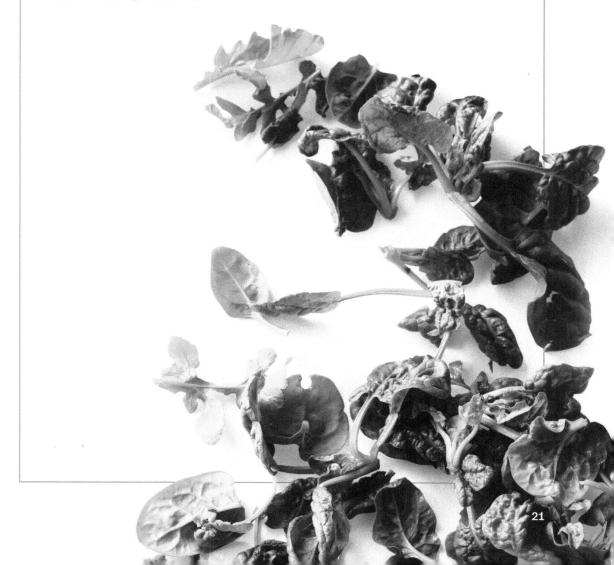

PART II

Treatment Plan

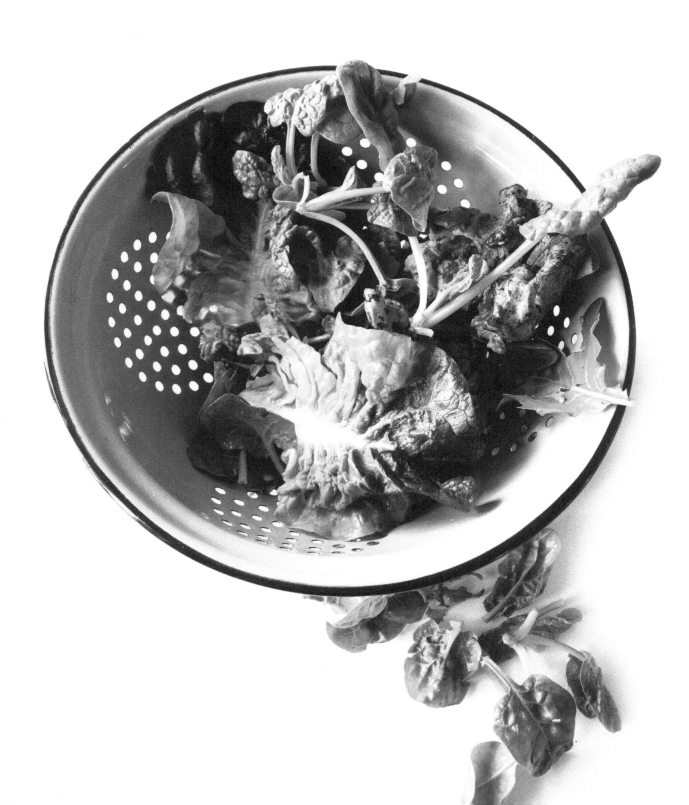

CHAPTER TWO

Holistic Changes
Make a Big Difference

Now that you have a better understanding of *Candida albicans*, what causes it to overgrow and become infectious, and the disastrous impacts this overgrowth can have on your body and overall well-being, you are ready to heal from the inside out. This chapter will give you the tools you need to be successful across the next few weeks while making your healing journey manageable for a busy lifestyle. Planning is often the key to success with any lifestyle change, so I strongly suggest spending a couple of days before beginning the program to prepare yourself for the coming weeks. The guidelines outlined in this chapter will provide you with a checklist for your preparation.

First Steps

Scheduling time for self-care is a big first step on the road to healing. Lifestyle change can be hard, and for many, this change will involve a big shift in dietary habits. I encourage you to make the weeks ahead as seamless and stress-free as possible by looking at other demands on your time such as social events, work commitments, and travel plans so that they do not derail your success. Planning meals ahead, identifying some convenience options for "on-the-go" days, and identifying some stress-relieving activities will be helpful in keeping you on track with your healing journey. Remember to be kind to your body as it heals: Get plenty of rest, reduce stress through relaxing and engaging in enjoyable activities, and include gentle exercise as you are physically able.

For many, a kitchen "cleanse" is a helpful first step to avoiding any potential temptations or gut-disturbing foods that could derail success. I recommend removing the items listed in the next section from your pantry, fridge, and freezer. Please note that there may be some overlap from one category to the next. For instance, salad dressing might be in the pantry or the refrigerator. What's important is if it's listed, please remove it. For individuals with family members or roommates who want to continue consuming these foods, you may want to place them in a designated area rather than getting rid of them altogether. However, for some, just knowing they are around will cause temptation, so it is important to have a conversation with these family members about the importance of dietary change for your (and their) overall health.

GET RID OF THE FOLLOWING . . .

PANTRY

- ☐ Baked goods, such as cookies or muffins
- ☐ Baking mixes, including pancake mixes
- ☐ Bars, such as granola or protein
- ☐ Beans, canned

- ☐ Breads and other grain products
- ☐ Candies
- ☐ Cereals, granolas, and flavored oatmeals
- ☐ Chips
- ☐ Cornstarch
- ☐ Crackers
- ☐ Drink mixes, including sugar-free or diet (such as cocoa, Crystal Light, MiO drops)
- ☐ Fruits, canned, dried (such as raisins), or other fruit snacks
- ☐ Marinara sauces and salsas that contain added sugar

- ☐ Nuts with added honey or sugars (such as honey roasted peanuts)
- ☐ Peanut butter, including flavored peanut butter
- ☐ Sugar, cane
- ☐ Sweeteners, both natural and artificial (including agave, honey, chocolate syrup, maple syrup, packets of artificial sweeteners, stevia and liquid stevia drops, and sugar alcohols such as erythritol, xylitol, and mannitol)
- ☐ Trail mixes that contain dried fruits, chocolates, peanuts, or yogurt

REFRIGERATOR

- ☐ Applesauce
- ☐ Beverages, artificially or sugar-sweetened (such as diet soda or "light" juice)
- ☐ Breads, such as canned biscuit dough or tortillas
- ☐ Condiments that contain added sugar, such as barbecue sauce, salad dressings, ketchup, marinades, sweet relish

- ☐ Fruit-based sweeteners, such as jams/jellies
- ☐ Jell-O (including sugar-free)
- ☐ Juices of any kind
- ☐ Milk, flavored creamers, and sweetened whipped cream
- ☐ Puddings
- ☐ Yogurts, flavored

☐ Breads, rolls, or other baked products

☐ Cakes, cookies, doughs, and other desserts

☐ Frozen entrées or meals

☐ Frozen fruit with added sugar (unsweetened berries are okay)

☐ Ice creams, sorbets, ice pops, and other frozen treats

☐ Juice concentrates, such as orange or lemonade

☐ Frozen veggies with seasoning that contain sugar (such as glazed carrots)

Plan Your Week Ahead

→ Look at your calendar for upcoming social events, activities, and travel plans to make sure you have a plan for prepped meals and grab-and-go snack options.

→ Using the sample meal plans outlined in chapter 3 and the recipes in chapters 4 through 7, plan meals one week at a time.

→ Create a grocery list based on the recipes you chose to try each week.

→ Find a day to devote to grocery shopping and meal prep. You do not have to cook all of the meals in one day, but cleaning and chopping veggies, portioning out snacks or salad toppings, and precooking meats will save you valuable time during the week ahead. For example, grilling or roasting several servings of chicken or steak ahead of time will make throwing together a simple weeknight salad or veggie bowl a breeze.

Some people desire more variety in their meals than others. If you are satisfied with eating the same one or two breakfast items every day, there is no need to spend too much time planning breakfast meal ideas. Many of the recipes in chapters 4 through 7 serve 1 to 2, but doubling these and using leftovers throughout the week or freezing extra portions for a quick and easy reheat meal can save time during a busy week. It is important to make this plan work for your lifestyle and cooking preferences to help reduce stress and maintain your focus on healing your body from the inside out.

Introduce Gentle Exercise

Your primary focus across the next few weeks will be on dietary changes to kill off candida overgrowth and infection and promote healing. For individuals not currently participating in a physical activity routine, this may not be the best time to start if you are feeling weak or physical symptoms from candidiasis preclude you from much activity. While gentle exercise can be helpful for ridding the body of toxins through lymphatic drainage and promoting stress reduction through the release of endorphins, incorporating exercise into the next few weeks should not be a source of any additional stress. Remember, your focus is on nutrition and healing.

For those who already incorporate physical activity into their regular lifestyle, there is no reason to stop this routine while undergoing the Natural Candida Cleanse dietary protocol. All activities you are currently doing are entirely appropriate to continue. However, when *Candida* start to die off, some individuals may find themselves feeling more fatigued or lacking motivation for regular activity. That is okay! Listen to your body and only incorporate the following activities if you are ready:

→ Biking or rowing
→ Resistance band exercises
→ Stretching or yoga exercises
→ Swimming
→ Walking, hiking, or light jogging

Allow for Rest and Adequate Sleep

Candidiasis and its associated symptoms can be exhausting, both mentally and physically. In order for our bodies to properly heal, we must give them the rest they need. I often give my clients the following analogy: If you pull your car into the driveway every evening and leave the motor running until you hop back in the next morning to head off again, that car isn't going to last very long. Not only are you going to run out of gas pretty quickly, but your car won't be as fuel-efficient and your engine will have a shorter life span. Why would we expect any other outcome from our bodies if we don't provide the essential rest that every cell needs for healing and proper function? Additionally, lack of sleep elevates blood glucose levels, which can deter candida die-off. In a fast-paced world, getting seven to eight hours of sleep a night may seem unlikely, but I encourage you to make this a goal throughout the weeks ahead.

Kitchen Essentials

Most of the recipes found in chapters 4 through 7 are designed for the novice cook and do not require many tools that are not already found in the average kitchen. However, there are some kitchen gadgets I find essential when embarking on a whole foods–based diet and making delicious and gut-healthy meals come together in a flash. I recommend that you invest in the following:

→ **Slow cooker or Instant Pot®:** Both are great tools that allow for hands-off cooking and save time in the kitchen. While the Instant Pot allows for last-minute meals, it can be a more expensive option. A traditional slow cooker or Crock–Pot takes a little more advanced planning (meals typically cook for four to six hours) but requires minimal prep and is 100 percent hands-off cooking that can be done even while you are away from the house. You can purchase a six- to eight-quart slow cooker for less than $30.

→ **Immersion blender or stand blender:** These are great for making smoothies, dressings, sauces, and soups. A blender is essential for homemade and gut-healthy versions of store-bought (and sugar-filled) staples. I prefer an immersion blender because it is affordable, versatile, and easy to clean! You can purchase one that can perform a variety of tasks for less than $30.

→ **Spiralizer:** This is a wonderful addition to a grain-free kitchen! You can get creative with a variety of vegetables to create "zoodles" and other pasta-free versions of old favorites. Many grocery stores now offer prepared spiralized veggies in the refrigerated produce section, but spending two minutes making these yourself will save you money in the long run. You can purchase a simple spiralizer for less than $20.

→ **Variety of storage containers for the refrigerator and freezer:** Glass or BPA-free plastic is preferred. Storing pre-chopped veggies or washed berries in the fridge for an easy grab-and-go snack or quick stir-fry will be a lifesaver midweek when life gets hectic. I also encourage you to consider doubling some recipes to freeze additional meals for when life throws you a curveball. Meetings run late or traffic puts us behind, and coming home to a frozen homemade meal that just needs reheated can be a very welcome reward for a few extra minutes spent in the kitchen.

→ **Insulated lunch bag and water bottle:** You will be packing your lunches and snacks daily to avoid processed and fast foods. Make it fun with a new lunch tote that can keep foods cold on longer car rides or days out and about. Water is essential to health and detoxification, so you will want to carry a water bottle with you to make sure you keep your fluids up!

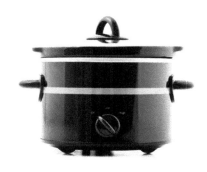

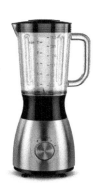

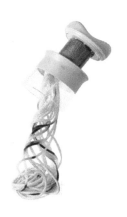

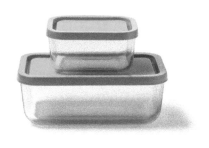

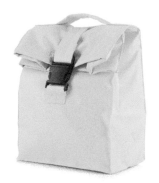

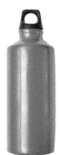

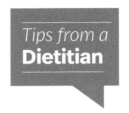

For most people, change is hard. Changing your dietary habits and routine can be challenging. If you are reading this book, you have likely tried many other interventions to relieve your symptoms and discomfort, but to no avail. You are up for the challenge! However, it is still important to remember that making changes often takes us out of our comfort zone, and I find that embracing this change and "being uncomfortable" from the start helps my clients be successful with following the Natural Candida Cleanse. A little more planning or prep time may be required to make sure you have delicious meal and snack options to avoid giving in to last-minute cravings. For many, giving up some favorite sweet treats, carb-heavy snacks, and convenience meals that may be comfort foods or part of a daily pattern will also be necessary. Rest assured that the initial small sacrifices are worth it! Remembering your goals and the end prize of digestive relief and improved health will help make this process easier. I encourage you to keep a journal throughout your healing journey to help process some of these changes and keep your focus on the end goal. For example, if you are used to having a sweet treat after dinner every night, the first couple of days of avoiding this will be a challenge for you. Feeling uncomfortable with this change is okay! You may journal about how hard saying no to that treat is and how you do not like it. But you have a powerful reason for doing so, and making positive steps toward your recovery is worth the sacrifice. You can wake up the next morning and journal about how proud of yourself you are for resisting that temptation and how much better you are feeling without the inflammation and gut disruption that sugary foods cause. You survived the challenge, and tonight, when it comes up again, you will be ready to confront and beat it again. Self-reflection and positive reinforcement exercises provide a vital level of emotional support that's integral to self-care and lifestyle change.

The Good, the Bad, and the Probiotics

Bacteria get a bad rap! We tend to think all bacteria are bad and cause illness. It's true that bacteria such as salmonella, staphylococcus, listeria, E-coli, and botulism enter our body through contaminated foods and environmental toxins. These bacteria can cause damage to our cells and tissues and can leave us very sick. However, our microbiome is quite varied and contains a lot of good bacteria that keep us healthy. As discussed in chapter 1 (see "Understanding Candida Overgrowth," page 4), a healthy microbiome is imperative to disease prevention, neurological health, gastrointestinal health, immunity, and overall wellness.

An overwhelming majority of the bacteria found in our digestive tract, genitourinary tract, skin, and mouth is not harmful and is actually considered vital for life. Good bacteria help us digest food and absorb nutrients, providing immunity and keeping us healthy and happy. A healthy microbiome is made up of about 80 to 85 percent beneficial bacteria in order to keep the other 15 to 20 percent of bad bacteria from harming us. When that balance becomes disrupted, gut dysbiosis is the result and can cause a host of complications. Candida overgrowth is one result of such imbalance. Candidiasis is a fungal infection caused by *Candida albicans* yeast.[9] It takes advantage of an unbalanced microbiome to overpower and cause inflammation and disease.

What about probiotics? These are examples of good bacteria found in foods and supplements that help promote a balanced microbiome and reverse gut dysbiosis. They are an essential part of the Natural Candida Cleanse because they restore balance and help defend the body against the invasive *Candida*. For this reason, I include fermented foods such as sauerkraut, kimchi, whole milk plain yogurt, and kefir in the Two-Week Natural Candida Cleanse outlined in the next chapter (page 47). Many of the bacteria shown to be beneficial in fighting candida infection are found in these foods.[10] However, additional probiotic supplementation is often necessary to fight candidiasis and ensure the return of healthy gut function.

A variety of different strains of bacteria (at least 10 to 20) ensures comprehensive therapeutic treatment. Some of the strains that are particularly beneficial in fighting candidiasis include: Lactobacillus rhamnosus, L. reuteri, L. acidophilus, L. lactis, L. helveticus, L. casei, Bifidobacterium breve, and B. bifidum.[11] Probiotics are also labeled with their concentration, or colony forming units (CFUs), of live and active bacteria cells. The higher the concentration, the more powerful the supplement. Look for brands with not only a variety of different strains of bacteria but also concentrations ranging from 35 to 90 billion CFUs. Refrigerated probiotics are not necessary, as there are many quality shelf-stable brands that retain their potency for up to two years.

What Happens When Bacteria Die in the Body?

A common side effect of beginning any therapeutic protocol that uses dietary intervention, probiotics, and/or antifungals to fight infectious candida overgrowth is die-off, also known as the Jarisch–Herxheimer reaction. Symptoms may get worse before they get better, and this is a natural part of the healing process. As the candida cells are starved or killed off by the introduction of probiotics and/or antifungals, they release a variety of endotoxins that cause inflammation and adverse effects. Common symptoms of die-off include headaches, GI complications (such as diarrhea, bloating, gas, and nausea), skin rashes, joint pain, brain fog, excessive sweating, and sometimes fever. These almost mimic the symptoms of candidiasis, so individuals often believe the treatment is not working for them. Hang in there! While your symptoms may temporarily get worse a few days into the Natural Candida Cleanse, they should resolve within the first week. If symptoms are severe, the Candida may be dying off more rapidly than your body can detoxify you, and you may need to back off on probiotic or antifungal use. I also encourage increased water intake, saunas or hot baths, dry skin brushing or exfoliating, and light exercise to help the body detoxify and rid itself of these endotoxins.

Understanding the Connection between Candida and Food

One of the main contributing factors to candida overgrowth is poor diet. Americans consume an overwhelming amount of processed foods, refined carbohydrates, and sugars. The fact that candidiasis affects so many people is no surprise. Fortunately, changing our dietary habits is 100 percent within our control. This lifestyle change is not always easy and requires dedication and determination. I have helped countless patients achieve success through diet and lifestyle change and create long-term solutions for health.

Candida albicans thrives on glucose from sugary and processed foods but can also receive a steady supply of food to stay alive and multiply from "healthy" carbohydrates. All carbohydrates contain glucose or can break down into glucose in your body. Fruits, whole grains, starchy vegetables and legumes, as well as "natural" sweeteners such as honey, maple syrup, and agave all provide food for the growing and thriving infectious candida colony. That is why the Natural Candida Cleanse eliminates all these foods for a finite period to starve off the *Candida* and restore microbiome balance and health. Some individuals may be able to reintroduce these foods in moderation following the treatment plan, but others prefer to only consume carbohydrates sparingly as they find they feel much better following a low-carbohydrate diet. I will further discuss a dietary approach to maintaining microbiome balance in chapter 3 (see "Naturopathic Healing," page 56).

Conversely, the nutrients in healthy fats and quality proteins do not break down into glucose. Instead, they serve to nourish your body and provide you with energy without supplying the *Candida* with fuel for life. I also promote a higher healthy-fat dietary approach in my Natural Candida Cleanse because I find these foods provide incredible satiety and make adherence to a lower-carbohydrate diet entirely sustainable. My patients often remark that they are amazed they do not miss some of their old favorite carbohydrate-rich foods such as breads, pastas, and rice because they are so satisfied with the complex flavors and filling nature of the foods included in the treatment plan. It is important to take a glass-half-full approach to dietary change. Rather than focusing on the foods you are eliminating from your diet, explore and embrace all the wonderful foods you can enjoy at every meal. You should not feel hungry at any point during your journey on the Natural Candida Cleanse. If you do, you need to include more of the foods from the "Foods to Enjoy" table (page 36). Remember, you are starving your candida overgrowth, not your body!

You will not be eliminating carbohydrates altogether, but rather getting them from lower-starch vegetables, low-sugar fruits, and some dairy (if including dairy in one's diet). These nutrient-dense vegetables and low-sugar fruits are rich in *phytochemicals*, the naturally occurring compounds found in plants that have amazing health benefits. Research strongly suggests that they play a role in disease prevention.[12] Additionally, many individuals with candida overgrowth experience various nutritional deficiencies due to malabsorption caused by a compromised GI tract. Low levels of vitamin B_{12}, iron, and the fat-soluble vitamins A, D, E, and K are common, making the inclusion of these nutrient-rich foods so important for healing.[13] Bottom line: Eat the veggies outlined in the following table to your heart's content to supply your body with a multitude of essential vitamins, minerals, and antioxidants for improved health, energy, and restored nutrient balance.

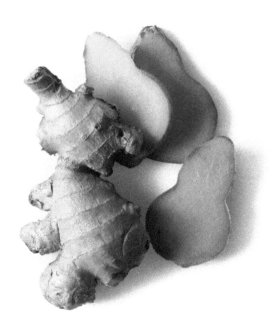

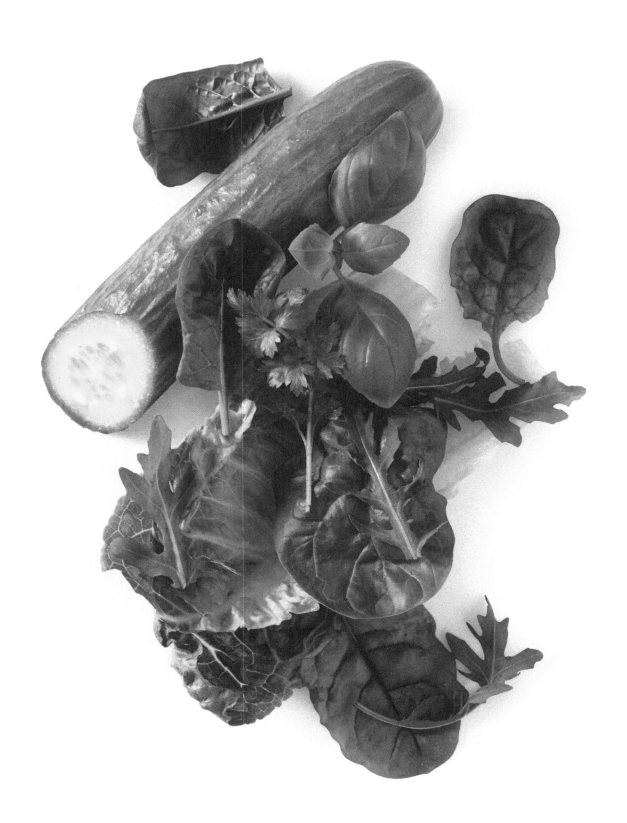

Foods to Enjoy

FOOD NAME	EXAMPLES	BENEFITS
⊘ Bone broth	Organic poultry or beef	→ High in collagen to restore gut lining integrity and help reverse leaky gut → Good source of protein for satiety
⊘ Citrus and low-sugar berries	Blackberries, blueberries, clementine (limit to one per day), lemon, lime, raspberries, strawberries	→ Darker berries are high in antioxidants → Great source of vitamin C for immunity
⊘ Coffee (in moderation)	Organic beans; limit to 12 ounces per day	→ For regular coffee drinkers, there is no need to battle going cold turkey during the Natural Candida Cleanse. However, coffee can be irritating to the stomach lining, hence the 12-ounce limit. Ideally any coffee you consume should be brewed from organic and well-sourced beans.
⊘ Limited dairy*	Goat cheese*, full-fat hard cheese, heavy cream*, full-fat cream cheese, whole milk kefir, organic whole milk plain yogurt (Greek)	→ Probiotics in fermented dairy for restoring healthy microbiome → Satiating and good source of protein
⊘ Healthy fats	Olives and olive oil, avocados and avocado oil, coconut and coconut oil, grass-fed butter*	→ Rich in anti-inflammatory omega-3 fatty acids → Provides satiety to reduce cravings
⊘ Fermented foods	Sauerkraut and kimchi	→ Probiotics to restore healthy microbiome and digestive comfort and regularity → High in fiber

* Note: Asterisk (*) represents a limited dairy suggestion. →

FOOD NAME	EXAMPLES	BENEFITS
⊘ Fresh herbs and spices	Allspice, cilantro, cinnamon, cumin, curry blends, ground ginger, mint, oregano, parsley, rosemary	→ Great sources of antioxidants and naturally detoxifying phytochemicals → Add variety and flavor to dishes
⊘ Quality proteins	Grass-fed beef, bison, and lamb; free-range eggs; liver and organ meats; antibiotic- and hormone-free pork; free-range poultry; wild-caught seafood	→ Well-sourced meats, seafoods, and animal products not raised on inflammatory corn or soy feed provide essential protein, vitamin B_{12}, iron, and other micronutrients to repair cell damage, provide energy, and allow the body to heal properly
⊘ Seeds, tree nuts	Flax, chia, hemp, pumpkin, sesame, almonds, walnuts, pecans, macadamia, Brazil nuts, hazelnuts	→ Rich in anti-inflammatory omega-3 fatty acids as well as essential vitamins and minerals → High in fiber to encourage elimination
⊘ Teas	Black, herbal, green	→ High in flavonoids, antioxidants that help protect cells from damage → Can help manage cravings → Black tea has antifungal properties to help kill off infection → Peppermint and ginger herbal teas can help with digestion

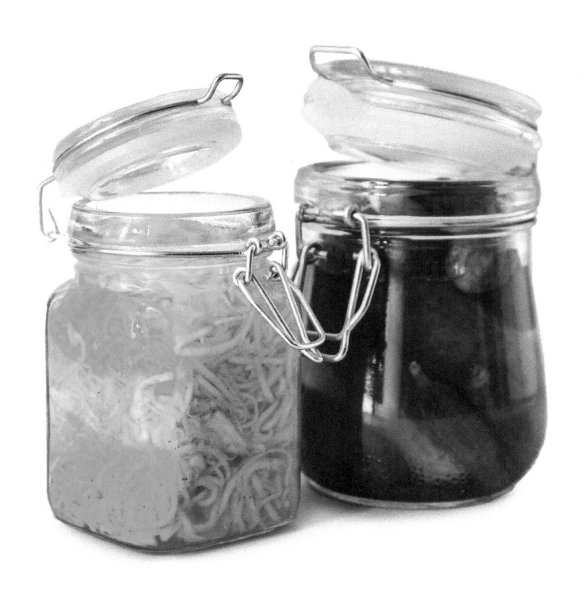

FOOD NAME	EXAMPLES	BENEFITS
✓ Cruciferous vegetables	Arugula, broccoli, Brussels sprouts, cabbage, cauliflower, collards, kale, rutabaga, radish, turnips	→ Contain sulforaphane, a phytochemical that assists in detoxification → Rich in antioxidants and micronutrients zinc and vitamins A, B, C, D, and E
✓ Non-starchy vegetables	Carrots, celery, cucumber, eggplant, jicama, bell peppers, spinach, tomatoes, zucchini, yellow squash	→ Colorful vegetables are rich in antioxidant carotenoids (precursors to vitamin A), such as beta carotene, lycopene, and lutein, that prevent cell damage → High levels of vitamin C to provide immunity by attacking free radicals in the body

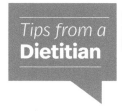

Tips from a
Dietitian

A Note on Dairy: Many of my patients do not experience adverse effects from including small amounts of low-lactose or fermented dairy products during or after the Natural Candida Cleanse. I include small amounts of certain dairy products in the plan because I find dairy to be a satiating source of probiotics, protein, fat, calcium, and potassium. In addition, it adds variety and flavor to many dishes. However, if you have trouble digesting dairy or find that it exacerbates symptoms, you can avoid it entirely during the program.

The following are serving-size suggestions for low-lactose, whole milk/full-fat dairy:

→ 1 tablespoon grass-fed butter

→ 1 ounce full-fat hard cheese (Cheddar, Parmesan, Swiss)

→ 2 tablespoons full-fat cream cheese (preferably grass-fed)

→ 1 tablespoon heavy cream

→ ½ cup whole milk plain kefir

→ ½ cup whole milk plain yogurt (preferably grass-fed)

Foods to Avoid

FOOD NAME	EXAMPLES	NEGATIVE EFFECTS
⊗ Alcohol	Beer, cider, spirits, wine	→ Inflammatory and can contribute to the deterioration of the gut lining, resulting in leaky gut syndrome → Can kill off good bacteria → Often leads to increased sugar cravings → Fermented alcohol contains yeast and/or fungi
⊗ Sweetened beverages	"Diet" drinks sweetened with artificial sweeteners or sugar alcohols, juices, kombucha, sodas, sweet teas	→ Feeds *Candida* → Diet drinks contain artificial sweeteners that contribute to gut dysbiosis and increase sugar cravings
⊗ Many dairy products	Most cheeses, cottage cheese, ice cream, milk (skim, 2%, whole)	→ Low-fat dairy contains higher levels of lactose, the naturally occurring sugar in milk, which feeds *Candida* → Can cause digestive discomfort in some individuals
⊗ High-sugar fruits	Apple, banana, cherry, grape, kiwi, mango, papaya, pear, pineapple	→ Naturally occurring fructose and glucose will feed *Candida*
⊗ Fungi and yeast products	Baked goods, beer, mushrooms, nutritional yeast flakes	→ Contributes to *Candida* overgrowth and infection
⊗ Grains (even "healthy" ones)	Barley, KAMUT®, oats, pasta, whole-wheat pasta, quinoa, rice, brown rice	→ Even gluten-free whole grains contain high levels of carbohydrates that will only feed *Candida*

FOOD NAME	EXAMPLES	NEGATIVE EFFECTS
⊗ Legumes	Beans (including chickpeas), lentils, peanuts	→ High in starch, which converts to glucose and provides food for candida growth → Pro-inflammatory
⊗ Milk	Skim milk, 1%, 2%, whole	→ Highly inflammatory and often difficult to digest → High in lactose, a naturally occurring milk sugar that can feed *Candida*
⊗ Refined vegetable oils	Canola, corn, cottonseed, soybean, sunflower	→ High in omega-6 fatty acids, which can be pro-inflammatory when consumed in excess
⊗ All processed and "boxed" foods	Cereals, chips, crackers	→ Even gluten-free versions of these foods contain high levels of carbohydrates, sugars, and other additives
⊗ Sugars and other "natural" sweeteners	Found in numerous processed foods such as cakes, fruit juices, muffins, and so on. Includes agave, honey, maple syrup, Stevia In The Raw®, etc.	→ Contributes to inflammation → Suppresses the immune system → Feeds *Candida*
⊗ Sugar substitutes	Aspartame, Splenda, stevia (okay in moderation if needed), sugar alcohols (erythritol, mannitol, xylitol)	→ Irritating to the gut lining → Can kill off good bacteria → Increases sugar cravings
⊗ High-starch veggies	Corn, potato, sweet potato, winter squash (acorn, butternut, spaghetti)	→ High starch converts rapidly to glucose in the body, which feeds *Candida*

How to Get the Most Out of Safe Foods

Remember, we are not only the plants or animals we eat but what they themselves were exposed to or ate as well. Therefore, it is so important to focus on not only gut-friendly and anti-inflammatory foods during this process but also on the *quality* of those same foods. The heavy commercialization of meat, poultry, and seafood production has led to the introduction of antibiotics, hormones, corn and soy feed, and often unsustainable harvesting practices. These additives and inflammatory agents are stored in the fat and protein of the animal or fish and get transferred to you when you consume them. I always recommend aiming for quality over quantity when it comes to protein sources. Most people can only absorb the amino acids from the protein in about 3 to 4 ounces of meat, fish, or poultry per meal, making a 6- to 8-ounce serving size excessive. If budget is a concern, as it is for most, I encourage you to aim for smaller amounts of higher-quality animal and fish protein sources. Look for grass-fed (and finished) meats, free-range and antibiotic- and hormone-free poultry and pork, and wild-caught seafood. Thankfully, as awareness mounts about the health benefits of quality protein sources, these products are becoming more and more mainstream and prices are coming down.

Remember that low-starch vegetables and low-sugar fruits are your friends! Full of essential micronutrients such as vitamins, minerals, and antioxidants, these powerhouses will help your body heal, restore nutrient balance, and provide energy. The more color, the better, so eat the rainbow! Much like our protein sources, many plant foods have been relegated to mass production and are exposed to pesticides and other harmful additives in the cultivation process. Organic or locally produced is always better, but if organic is not always an option, a good rule of thumb is that if you are going to eat the peel, buy organic. If not, conventional is a good second option. For example, conventionally produced avocados and citrus (unless using a lemon or lime for zesting) would be fine to use, whereas berries and salad greens are best to buy organic. Additionally, foods that grow in the ground absorb all of the runoff from pesticide and other sprays, making root vegetables such as carrots, parsnips, turnips, and rutabagas even more susceptible to contamination.

Be sure to reference the Dirty Dozen list (see page 141) for a complete list of fruits and vegetables to always buy organic if possible.

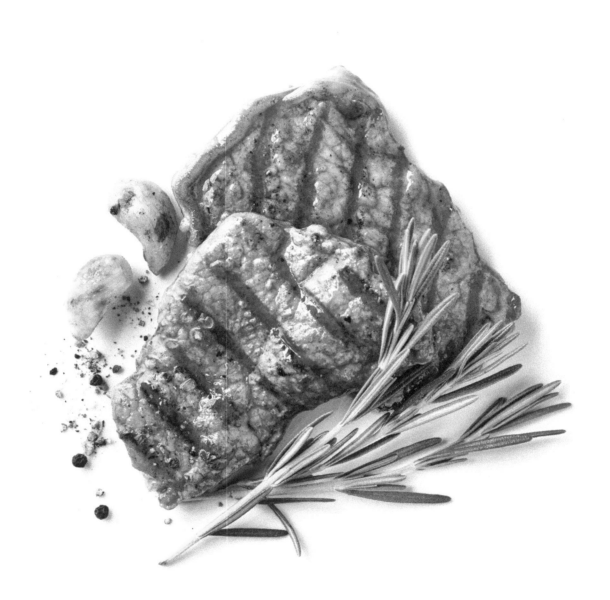

CASE STUDY

When I provided Lisa an outline of my dietary protocol to rid her body of the *Candida* that had taken over and was causing her such distress, she was worried it would be too overwhelming for her. After all, she was used to frequent "healthy" convenience options and did not like to spend too much time in the kitchen. She felt at a loss as to what she would even eat for lunch if it could not be a sandwich from her favorite local deli. We spent some time looking at her week ahead, assessing her time commitments, including work meetings and dinner with a friend. We went over the list of safe foods and identified all the ones she was really excited about and went through a handful of quick and easy recipes that she could make in bulk so she'd have leftovers for lunch the next day and even a few portions to freeze for the following week. We found the menu online for the restaurant where Lisa would be dining with her friend and made some selections that would be safe for her to enjoy. Lisa really enjoyed working in her garden for exercise and stress relief, and since the weather was getting nice, we made a plan for projects outdoors in the weeks ahead. She left my office feeling confident and ready to begin her healing process.

At our first follow-up appointment one week later, Lisa admitted to feeling better overall than she had the week prior but reported that the first few days were pretty rough for her. She did not feel as great one week out as she had hoped. She had experienced headaches that started in the late afternoon and persisted into the evening almost daily, and her energy seemed even lower than it had in months previous, which she did not think was possible. The headaches were gone, but she was still lacking energy. I reminded her of the common transition period when beginning the protocol and assured her that her symptoms were likely due to a combination of sugar and refined carbohydrate withdrawal, as well as *Candida* die-off and the release of endotoxins into her system. She admitted she had not been drinking as much water and just did not have the energy to get out to her garden but would work on incorporating both going forward. I decreased her probiotic supplement to a half dose until the end of the protocol but encouraged her to continue with the probiotic foods she was including in her diet. As a last bit of encouragement, I reminded her that these symptoms she was feeling were signs her body was fighting off the *Candida* and starting its road toward healing and that this period was only temporary. She was optimistic and determined to continue with her journey.

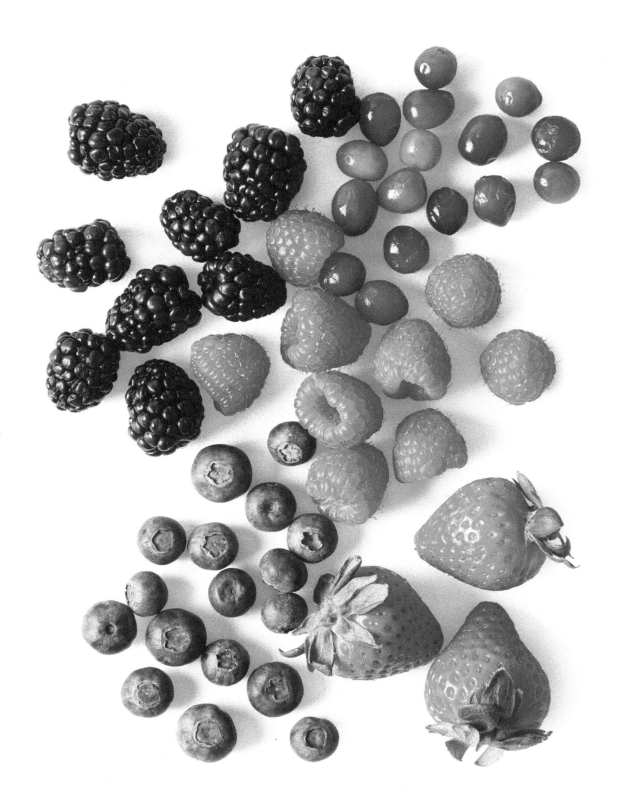

CHAPTER THREE

The Natural
Candida Cleanse

Now that you have spent some time preparing yourself both mentally and physically for the weeks ahead, you are ready to embark on your journey to better health! Remember that the first few days may present some challenges, but the result is well worth the commitment to the process. This chapter outlines the Natural Candida Cleanse and provides some sample meal plans to get you started, as well as support to coach you through the potential and natural challenges of lifestyle change. Recipes for flavorful, satiating, and varied meals are found in chapters 4 through 7. Now let's get started!

Grocery List

The following grocery list is a great starting point to load up your kitchen with some basics for grab-and-go snacks, quick meals, and many of the ingredients found in the recipes in the following chapters. It is meant to serve as a guide for providing some variety. If you do not enjoy or have intolerances to any of the following foods, please feel free to omit them in your personalized plan.

STOCK UP ON . . .

PANTRY

- ☐ Bone broth (chicken or beef)
- ☐ Unsweetened almond or sunflower butter
- ☐ Unsweetened cocoa
- ☐ Unsweetened flaked coconut
- ☐ Almond flour, coconut flour
- ☐ Nuts: almonds, walnuts, pecans, macadamia, hazelnuts, Brazil nuts
- ☐ Olive oil, avocado oil, coconut oil, sesame oil
- ☐ Canned sauerkraut
- ☐ Canned seafood: tuna, salmon, sardines, anchovies
- ☐ Seltzer waters with no natural or artificial sweeteners
- ☐ Spices such as cinnamon, allspice, pumpkin pie spice (no sugar added), ground ginger, cumin, chili powder, garlic powder, onion powder, curry blends
- ☐ Tamari
- ☐ Teas: herbal, black, and green (no sugar added)
- ☐ Canned tomatoes: diced and puréed (no sugar added)
- ☐ Apple cider vinegar

REFRIGERATOR

- ☐ Cooking aromatics such as garlic, fresh ginger, leeks, and green onions
- ☐ Avocados
- ☐ Grass-fed butter

- ☐ Capers

- ☐ Goat cheese

- ☐ Citrus such as clementine, lemon, and lime

- ☐ Fermented dairy such as plain whole milk Greek yogurt, whole milk kefir

- ☐ Eggs (preferably free-range)

- ☐ Salad greens such as arugula, endive, kale, baby lettuces, romaine lettuce, and spinach

- ☐ Olives

- ☐ Fresh veggies for snacking such as broccoli, carrots, cauliflower, cucumber, jicama, bell peppers, radishes, snow peas, and cherry tomatoes

FREEZER

- ☐ Frozen berries such as blackberries, blueberries, raspberries, and strawberries

- ☐ Seeds: chia, flax, hemp, pumpkin, sesame (store in freezer to keep fresh)

- ☐ Frozen veggies such as asparagus, broccoli, green beans, Brussels sprouts, cauliflower, bell peppers, spinach, green and yellow squash (avoid vegetable blends containing beans, corn, mushrooms, peas, and potatoes)

Two-Week Natural Candida Cleanse

This program is designed to rid your body of damaging candida overgrowth by starving the existing infectious Candida, restoring gut health and a balanced microbiome with naturally healing and nutrient-dense foods, and setting you up for long-term success with a new approach to nutrition and lifestyle habits. For many, complete relief from symptoms can be accomplished by following the Natural Candida Cleanse for just two weeks. Everyone suffering from candida overgrowth will experience some reduction in their symptoms after just two weeks of following the protocol, provided the symptoms are not the result of an unrelated underlying condition or complication. The duration of your treatment will depend on the severity of your candidiasis and how well you comply with the dietary protocol. In this chapter, I will discuss some circumstances that may require a longer treatment.

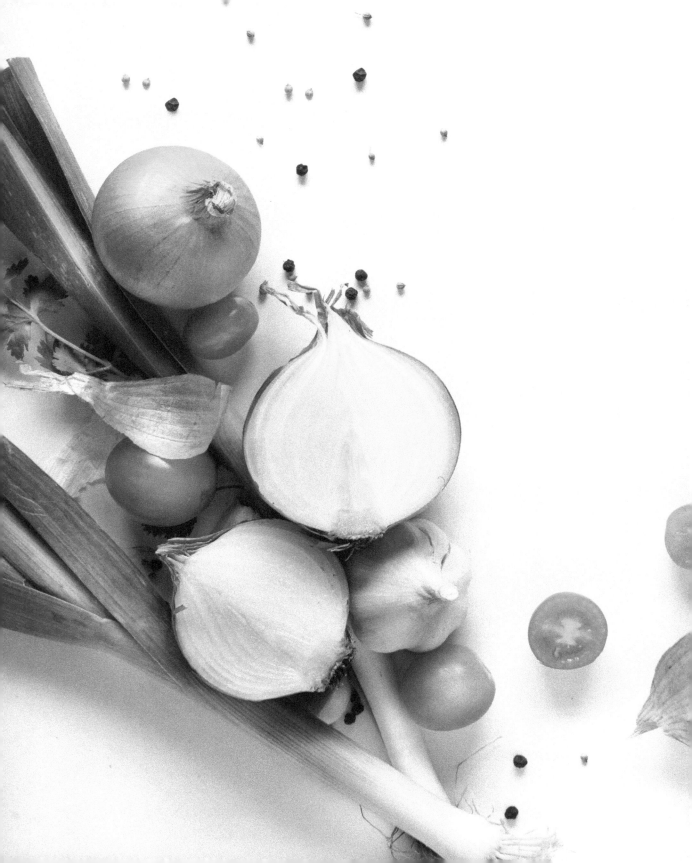

My patients often ask me about a "cleanse" or "detox" to jump-start their journey. I do not believe that a short-term "detox" is necessary nor effective. In fact, often, a period of extreme restriction only results in feelings of deprivation and increased frustration. On top of that, our bodies are equipped with a naturally detoxifying system! We have a liver, kidneys, lungs, and a lymphatic system that, when given the proper nutrition, are 100 percent effective at detoxifying our bodies every day. In this chapter, I will also outline tips for maximizing this detoxification process, including nutrition, hydration, and light exercise.

The Natural Candida Cleanse is designed to be effective while still allowing you to enjoy flavorful and satiating foods without any caloric restriction. Remember that food is medicine and we are what we eat. While you may be able to resume eating some of the foods that are eliminated in the Natural Candida Cleanse, you should use these next two weeks to not only rid your body of candida overgrowth but also commit to healthy lifestyle and dietary changes for long-term success.

WHAT HAPPENS IN THIS PROCESS?

By eliminating all sugars, refined carbohydrates, processed foods, whole grains, starchy vegetables, high-sugar fruits, and low-fat dairy, you drastically reduce your glucose and intake of other carbohydrates, thus cutting off the food supply to invasive Candida. As they starve and begin to die off, we sometimes see a brief worsening of symptoms due to the release of endotoxins (see "What Happens When Bacteria Die in the Body?" page 32). This can make the first three to four days of the Natural Candida Cleanse challenging for many. I will discuss ways to help your body naturally detoxify in the sections that follow (see pages 52 to 55). Remember, symptoms of die-off are a good sign your body is on its way to recovery and healing.

Another challenge many find in the first few days of the Natural Candida Cleanse is combatting sugar cravings and the associated symptoms of sugar withdrawal. Sugar is addictive! It works on the same dopamine receptors in our brains as opioids and other addictive chemicals, and for someone who is used to frequently consuming foods high in sugars, breaking the cycle of addiction can be tricky. Here are some possible symptoms of sugar withdrawal and suggestions to help you cope during the first week:

Headaches: When you remove a foreign substance to which your body has become addicted, withdrawal headaches are common in the first two to three days. Combat these by increasing water intake to help flush out toxins and keep your brain and body hydrated. Aim for a minimum of 100 ounces per day.

Mood swings: Once your usual supply of sugar gets cut, your body may rebel with fluctuating moods and energy levels. Make sure to nourish yourself with high-quality proteins and healthy fat sources, as well as vitamins and minerals from colorful non-starchy vegetables, to keep yourself satiated and help flush out toxins.

Intense cravings: Here is that addictive cycle at work. Once you cut off the steady supply of straight glucose, your body will crave that "high," making you want to reach for sweets and other refined carbohydrates such as breads, chips, and crackers. Combat these cravings with more water, high-quality proteins, and healthy fats included in the "Foods to Enjoy" table (see page 36). Using lots of flavor in your cooking with herbs and spices will also help keep your palate satisfied without the usual dose of sugar. Light physical activity such as walking or biking will help your body rid itself of excess glucose faster as well and get you on the road to reduced cravings.

Water intake is so crucial for the natural detoxification process in your liver, kidneys, and lymphatic system. I recommend a minimum of 100 ounces (about 10 to 12 glasses) of water daily during the Natural Candida Cleanse protocol. For many, this can feel overwhelming, and if you are not used to consuming water regularly, you may find yourself running to the bathroom frequently. Again, that is a great sign your body is detoxifying! For those who have trouble keeping up with their water intake, I suggest trying the following strategies:

Cluster drinking: If sipping water regularly throughout the day does not work for your schedule or lifestyle, you can still achieve your daily water goals with less-frequent drinking. Start the day with 24 ounces of water first thing after waking. Have another 24 ounces before you eat lunch. Aim for another 24 when leaving work or just before sitting down to dinner. End your day with 24 ounces of water or herbal tea before bed.

Setting a timer or alarm: You can set an alarm on your phone or watch to go off every hour during the day to remind you to drink an 8- to 12-ounce glass of water. At the end of an 8-hour workday, you will have hit your goal!

Herbal teas and seltzer waters: Even the best water drinkers get tired of water some days. Herbal teas and unsweetened or naturally flavored seltzer waters also count toward your daily water goals. Alternatively, you can add a slice of lemon, lime, or orange to your water for some extra flavor. Caffeinated beverages such as black tea, green tea, and coffee are all-natural diuretics, meaning they contribute to dehydration rather than hydration, so while these are allowed in moderation on the Natural Candida Cleanse, I do not count these beverages toward water goals.

Mix up the temperature: Some people love their water ice-cold while others prefer room temperature. Make sure you are drinking water at the temperature you prefer. This simple change has helped increase water consumption in many of my patients.

Other ways to augment natural detoxification include:

→ Exercising lightly to help lymphatic drainage
→ Sweating from intense exercise or a sauna/steam room session
→ Body scrubbing with a hot, wet towel before or after a bath or shower

→ Dry skin brushing or exfoliation
→ Eating sulfur-rich foods such as cruciferous vegetables, garlic, and artichoke (see the "Foods to Enjoy" table, page 36)

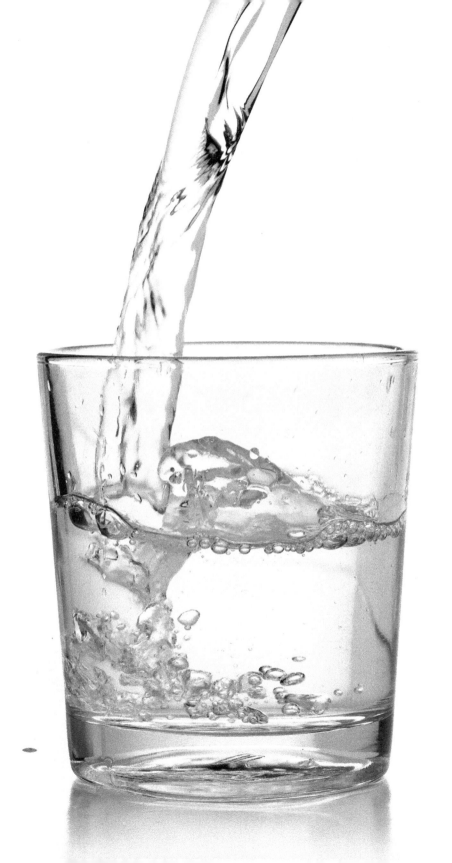

As your body detoxifies and rids itself of harmful candidiasis, the inclusion of probiotics through fermented foods and OTC supplementation, in combination with phytochemicals in the foods included in the meal plan, allows for the restoration of a healthy and balanced microbiome and digestive comfort. Additional healing may be needed for those with more invasive or longer-term candidiasis, and I recommend including collagen daily, either through bone broth or collagen powder, to restore and repair gut lining integrity.

Additional supplements can be helpful during the Natural Candida Cleanse:

L-glutamine: This amino acid vital to intestinal lining repair. I prefer the powder form. Two to five grams daily (about 1 teaspoon of powder) is recommended during the two-week program and beyond for gut health.

Zinc: Like L-glutamine, zinc helps strengthen intestinal wall lining. It also increases immunity. Take 50mg daily.

Vitamin A: This vitamin helps strengthen cell walls and can improve gut lining integrity. Take 10,000 IU daily.

Dandelion root tea: This tea has natural detoxifying properties. Can help tame carbohydrate and sugar cravings. Limit to 1 serving per day.

Digestive enzymes: These enzymes may help reduce bloating and gas after meals in some individuals. Will help ease the transition to a new way of eating for those not used to high amounts of healthy fats and/or animal proteins. Be sure to look for products that contain a variety of enzymes, including amalyse, lipase, and protease.

Multivitamin or B-complex: Many who suffer from long-term candidiasis are deficient in many essential micronutrients and may have trouble with malabsorption. Taking a multivitamin may also help with lower energy levels and improve immunity.

Naturopathic Healing

The Natural Candida Cleanse employs the naturopathic "4R" approach used in various healing modalities to successfully treat and manage a variety of conditions. To effectively cure candidiasis and prevent recurrence, four distinct therapies are often used simultaneously: REMOVE, REPLACE, REINOCULATE, and REPAIR. This method effectively supports each phase of treatment and promotes long-term health and success.

→ **Remove:** The Natural Candida Cleanse removes the foods that promote candida growth and infection. This causes starvation and die-off of the infectious microorganisms, which are then removed from your body via natural detoxification pathways.

→ **Replace:** Rather than simply removing foods from the diet, the Natural Candida Cleanse replaces these pro-candida foods with healthy fats and proteins that promote healing and digestive support without allowing the *Candida* to flourish.

→ **Reinoculate:** Restoring healthy microbiome balance is imperative for long-term health and the prevention of future candida overgrowth. The Natural Candida Cleanse includes a variety of probiotic-rich fermented foods, as well as those dense in nutrients, healing antioxidants, and immunity-building vitamins and minerals.

→ **Repair:** Leaky gut and intestinal permeability is so often associated with candida overgrowth (see "What Is Leaky Gut Syndrome?," page 11). Healing and strengthening the gut lining is essential to prevent relapse, promote healthy digestion, and avoid widespread inflammation.

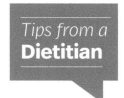

As you see from the "Foods to Enjoy" table (page 36), the sample meal plan (pages 58 to 59), and the list of recipes in chapters 4 through 7, I include a lot of animal and seafood protein in the Natural Candida Cleanse. Well-sourced, high-quality animal and seafood proteins are the most well-absorbed sources of essential amino acids for cell repair and healing. When I work with patients who follow a vegan or vegetarian diet, the first question I ask them is their reasoning behind that way of eating. While I understand many may abstain from animal and seafood proteins for moral or religious reasons, I stress the health benefits of including these in your diet, specifically when using dietary intervention to rid the body of candidiasis. Unfortunately, many of the sources of protein common in a vegetarian or vegan diet are also high in carbohydrates so they are foods that are not conducive to a candida cleanse (e.g., tofu, beans and legumes, many forms of dairy). It is possible to follow a vegetarian and/or vegan diet during the Natural Candida Cleanse, but proteins will be limited and there will be less variety in your meals. This is fine in the short-term, and after the two-week removing, replacing, reinoculating, and repairing treatment has concluded, reintroduction of soy and other starchier vegetarian proteins may be tolerated in moderation with continued success. I do not include a sample meal plan specifically for plant-based diets, but you are welcome to omit animal or seafood proteins as desired in many of the recipes that follow. I encourage you to speak with a registered dietitian or your trusted healthcare provider about ensuring that your protein needs are met if you follow the protocol for more than one month.

SAMPLE 2-WEEK MEAL PLAN

Tips to remember:

1 Start each morning with a minimum of 8 to 12 ounces of water to help with natural detoxification and reduced negative symptoms.

2 Snacks are optional and need to be included only if you feel hungry between meals. They are not limited to just once a day.

3 Your main focus is on avoiding the foods that feed and promote candida overgrowth (processed and packaged foods, sugars, carbohydrates, grains, high-sugar fruits, high-starch vegetables). If you need to include MORE of the safe foods listed in the "Foods to Enjoy" table on page 36, please do so. The following is simply a guide for two weeks' worth of meal ideas.

4 Recipes identified in this book as lunch recipes can be made for dinner, and dinner recipes can be made for lunch.

	BREAKFAST	LUNCH	DINNER	SNACK
DAY 1	Yogurt Parfait (page 72)	Healthy Fats Salad (page 83)	Spiced Meatballs in Coconut Curry over Cauliflower Rice (page 112)	Energy Balls (page 107)
DAY 2	Creamy Cauliflower "Oatmeal" (page 79)	Egg and Avocado Salad with Endive Spears (page 82)	Chicken Thighs with Creamy Arugula Pesto over Zucchini Noodles (page 114)	Energy Balls
DAY 3	Southwestern Egg Muffins (page 76)	Tarragon Chicken Salad (page 91)	Salmon Cakes with Asparagus Almondine (page 118)	Gut-Healing Chicken Soup (page 92)
DAY 4	Gut-Healing Green Smoothie (Dairy-Free) (page 106)	Cream of Cauliflower Soup (page 84)	Slow Cooker Greek Chicken with Cauliflower Tabouli (page 116)	Yogurt Parfait
DAY 5	Florentine Frittata (page 70)	Creamy Lime-Cilantro Tuna Salad (page 96)	Southwestern Stuffed Peppers (page 120)	Chocolate and Almond Chia Pudding (page 108)

	BREAKFAST	LUNCH	DINNER	SNACK
DAY **6**	Grain-Free Pancakes with Berry Sauce (page 78)	Almond Joy Smoothie (Dairy-Free) (page 102)	Slow Cooker Pork Carnitas in lettuce wraps** (page 129)	Energy Balls
DAY **7**	Baked Egg in Avocado (page 75)	Gut-Healing Chicken Soup	Slow Cooker Pork Carnitas over spinach salad with avocado**	Yogurt Parfait
DAY **8**	Southwestern Egg Muffins	Tarragon Chicken Salad with Seedy Crackers (pages 91 and 109)	Easy Marinara Sauce over Zoodles (pages 133 and 114)	Gut-Healing Chicken Soup
DAY **9**	Probiotic-Rich Blueberry Smoothie (page 103)	Healthy Fats Salad	Stir-Fried Beef and Broccoli (page 126)	Chocolate and Almond Chia Pudding
DAY **10**	Florentine Frittata	Almond Joy Smoothie	Coleslaw Salad with Shredded Rotisserie Chicken (page 88)	Gut-Healing Chicken Soup
DAY **11**	Creamy Cauliflower "Oatmeal"	Egg and Avocado Salad with Seedy Crackers (pages 82 and 109)	Spinach salad with pulled rotisserie chicken**	Gut-Healing Green Smoothie (Dairy-free)
DAY **12**	Baked Egg in Avocado	Creamy Lime-Cilantro Tuna Salad	Slow Cooker Pork Carnitas over Kale Salad with Lemon-Tahini Dressing (page 90)	Gut-Healing Chicken Soup
DAY **13**	Yogurt Parfait	Gut-Healing Chicken Soup	Sage and Citrus Roasted Pork Chops (page 121)	Energy Balls
DAY **14**	Avocado "Toast" (page 73)	Cream of Cauliflower Soup	Crispy Coconut Salmon (page 128)	Chocolate and Almond Chia Pudding

** Double asterisk denotes meals or parts of meals that are not included as recipes in this book. Rather, these are fill-ins, or ways to use convenience meals such as plain baby spinach, store-bought rotisserie chicken, canned tuna, etc.

Closing Words of Advice

I am so glad you have chosen to take control of your health and make some very impactful dietary and lifestyle changes that will allow you to find relief from the debilitating symptoms of candidiasis and heal your body from the inside out. The information in the previous chapters provides you with the education and understanding to truly be successful on this journey. You have spent time preparing yourself, both physically and mentally, for the weeks ahead, and I have faith that you are ready to get started.

I want to add another layer of support for some common pitfalls and questions I hear from my patients. Remember, keeping a journal throughout this process can be incredibly helpful for motivation and persistence, and I encourage you to do so. Even in the best of circumstances, challenges may arise. Do not get discouraged—these are a natural part of any lifestyle change, and you are not alone! Here are some tips to help you through possible challenges:

MY CRAVINGS ARE SO INTENSE

Sugar is addictive! On top of that, the infectious yeast signal you to crave more sugar and carbohydrate-rich foods so they can be fed. Cravings are not a result of being weak; rather, they are a very natural side effect of your condition. Know that the longer you resist giving in to your cravings, the less intense they will become, eventually disappearing completely. Some suggestions to help you through the first week:

Journal, journal, journal. Talk yourself through the craving, remind yourself of your goals and the end result, and make sure to journal how great it feels to NOT give in and know that you are making your body healthier and stronger.

Find an alternate activity. Remove yourself from the temptation, take a walk, listen to music, or take a hot bath.

Use warm herbal teas to break the evening sweet tooth cycle. If your nightly routine used to be grabbing something sweet before bed, replace this habit with a new evening tea routine.

Turn off the electronics. Often, sitting in front of the TV or computer is a trigger for negative eating patterns and simply removing this activity breaks the addictive cycle.

Remember that the goal is to avoid the foods that will inhibit die-off or lead to further overgrowth. You do not need to be concerned about an extra snack or an overly large portion of safe food. If that helps you overcome a craving and not consume candida-feeding foods, you are doing great. The first week can be difficult, so be kind to yourself and remember that you are working toward ridding your body of candida infection and all of the uncomfortable and debilitating symptoms that come with it. Don't put food on a pedestal: No sugary or starchy food TASTES better than BEING better feels!

WHAT TO DO IF I CHEAT?

Put it behind you and get right back to business! Often, we do not get derailed from success by an insular incident; rather, our cause is lost when we feel our efforts are hopeless. One cheat meal or food does not have to mean that the entire process needs to end. It is important to accept the cheat and move on by getting right back to the meal plan. It may require a longer duration to allow for your body to fully heal, but all efforts should not be abandoned. We are only human and none of us is perfect.

HOW TO HANDLE RESTAURANTS?

I suggest using the recipe and meal plan ideas to prepare as many of your meals at home as possible throughout the next two-week period. However, sometimes eating out is inevitable. If you have to eat out, do not be afraid to be picky! Ask your server details about food preparation and sauces if it is not clearly stated on the menu. Ask for dishes without the sauces and dressings, as these tend to be where sugars and other additives hide. Avoid breaded meats and fish, and load up on veggies if possible. If a restaurant meal is a necessity, make sure you don't arrive starving. It will be hard to resist chips, breads, and other carb-heavy fillers if you are ravenously hungry! Have a high-protein and/or healthy-fat snack (such as Energy Balls on page 107) an hour or two before your meal. Order a side salad to start if the table is loading up on carb-heavy appetizers so you won't feel left out. Drink your water!

WHAT ABOUT SUGAR SUBSTITUTES?

When asking anyone to eliminate sugar from their diet, I am constantly asked about sugar substitutes. While they may be a better alternative to the real deal because they won't feed *Candida* and other infectious micro-organisms, they are like putting a Band-Aid on a gunshot wound. Here's why: Nonnutritive sweeteners (e.g., Splenda, Truvia, or Equal) are 200 to 700 times sweeter than their "natural" counterpart. When we replace natural sugars (agave, honey, maple syrup, table sugar, and the like) with these substitutes, we don't train our taste buds to adapt to a less-sweet product. Rather, sugar substitutes tell them to crave even sweeter foods, making breaking the sugar addiction that much more difficult. While we may be decreasing the physiological addiction to sugar when we partake in substitutes, we aren't addressing the psychological component of the sweet craving. Sugar alcohols should be avoided on the Natural Candida Cleanse because they can cause bloating and diarrhea when consumed in excess, especially in individuals predisposed to food sensitivities and gut imbalance.

Bottom line: Sugar substitutes are okay to use on occasion in dessert recipes at the conclusion of the Natural Candida Cleanse protocol, but these foods should still be thought of as "treats" and not staples in your day-to-day diet. Moderation is always the best approach! At the end of the two weeks, you may not even have a desire for sweet foods anymore because you will have broken the addictive cycle and trained your taste buds to enjoy less-sweet flavors.

WHEN TO STOP THE NATURAL CANDIDA CLEANSE PROTOCOL AND SEE A PROFESSIONAL

While symptoms from Candida die-off are quite common and natural in the beginning stages of the Natural Candida Cleanse (see "What Happens When Bacteria Die in the Body?", page 32), developing new symptoms or symptoms that inhibit daily life should be a sign that it is time to see a trusted medical provider. These include the symptoms that were laid out in chapter 1 (see "When Is It Time/Safe to Take Matters into Your Own Hands?", page 16) and are repeated here:

→ Blood in stool or urine
→ Vomiting
→ Severe abdominal pain that is constant
→ Swelling in legs
→ Lightheadedness or feeling faint
→ Blurred vision

→ Tingling sensation in extremities
→ Severe thirst or frequent urination
→ Chest pain
→ Shortness of breath or trouble breathing

WHAT'S NEXT?

Once you have completed the Natural Candida Cleanse and the majority of your symptoms from candidiasis have disappeared, it is likely you have killed off most of the infectious *Candida*, your body has begun to heal itself, and your microbiome is on its way to being balanced and healthy once again. However, it is important to remember that to maintain symbiosis and optimal health, many of the dietary and lifestyle changes you have learned in this process should be continued going forward. The two-week protocol mandates a strict exclusion of most carbohydrate-containing but otherwise nutrient-dense foods such as many starchy vegetables, fruits, and whole grains. While I believe that everyone should endeavor to avoid added sugars, processed foods, and refined carbohydrates in their diet, including moderate amounts of nutrient- and fiber-dense carbohydrates can be part of a balanced and healthy lifestyle.

Tips for Long-Term Success

Nutrition guidelines should always be customized for individual needs and lifestyle and health concerns, but in general, I recommend adhering to these guidelines for long-term sustained success:

→ Avoid all processed and packaged foods (frozen entrées, "boxed" foods including crackers, chips, and cereals), refined carbohydrates or "white" foods (including most pasta, white rice, most store-bought breads, tortillas, and wraps), and all sweetened beverages (including soda and juice). Aim to limit added sugars to no more than 5 to 10 grams per day. These are found in otherwise "healthy" foods such as yogurt, salad dressing, salsas and sauces, and trail mixes. Label reading is key!

→ You can reintroduce starchier vegetables such as potatoes, sweet potatoes, and winter squash, legumes such as beans and lentils, as well as whole grains such as brown rice, oats, quinoa, and millet as tolerated, but limit your intake to a half-cup serving per meal.

→ Continue to include a variety of non-starchy vegetables, low-sugar fruits, quality protein sources, and healthy fats to make up the bulk of your meals.

→ Limit sweet "treats," including those using sugar substitutes, to no more than one per week, if at all.

→ Continue with your water intake. At this point, it should feel less overwhelming, and your body likely has adjusted to the added volume. This will also help you continue with the natural detoxification process that is ongoing.

→ If you feel you have strayed from your nutrition goals and your symptoms begin to return, adhere to the Natural Candida Cleanse for two weeks to restore balance.

Lisa came to our second follow-up appointment at the conclusion of her two weeks on my dietary protocol with a huge smile on her face. She reported drastically improved digestion and was thrilled to tell me she felt like a new woman. She no longer feared being in public after meals due to extreme bloating and gas and was seeing a lot of improvement in her skin irritations, which also brought her a renewed sense of confidence. Her energy had more than doubled in the past week, and, with improvements in her asthma, she was enjoying time in her garden as well as regular walks in the evenings after work. The best part? She loved the foods she was eating! After having previously restricted so many foods she believed were the sources of her problems and/or were "unhealthy," she considered her diet now to be the most varied it had been in over a year. She had no desire to go back to the carbohydrates and sugary foods she had been consuming. We discussed a transition plan, and Lisa decided to stay on the dietary protocol for another two weeks to ensure her recovery would be long-term. Her nail fungus persisted, but as she continued with antifungal creams, this too cleared up within the first month. Her transition plan included reintroducing small amounts of starchier vegetables on occasion but continuing to avoid foods with added sugars and gluten. She limited gluten-free whole grains to no more than a half-cup serving two times per week and continued to only consume lower-sugar fruits, as higher-sugar options tasted too sweet to her now. She continued taking an OTC probiotic supplement and incorporating fermented foods into her meals three to four times per week.

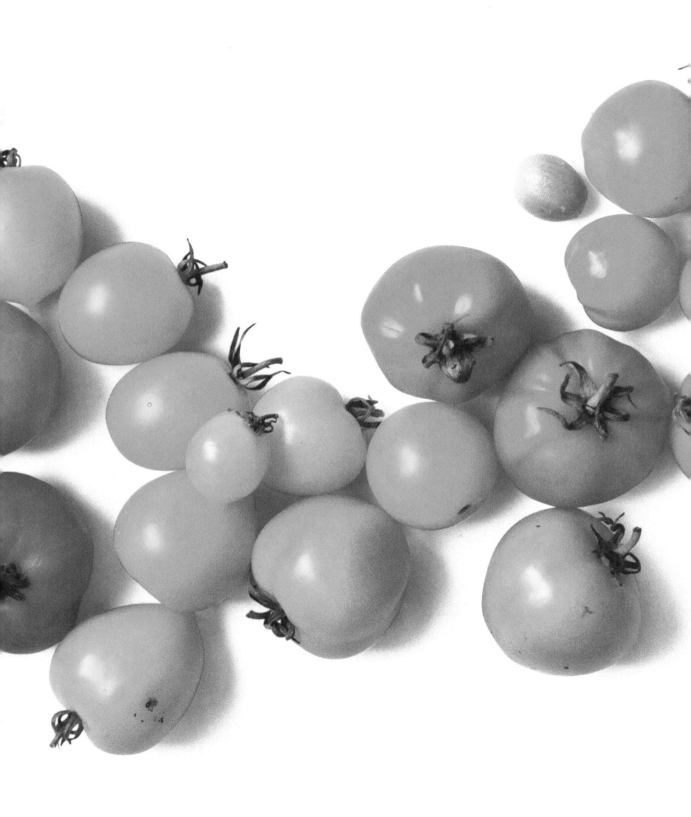

PART III

Treatment Plan
Recipes

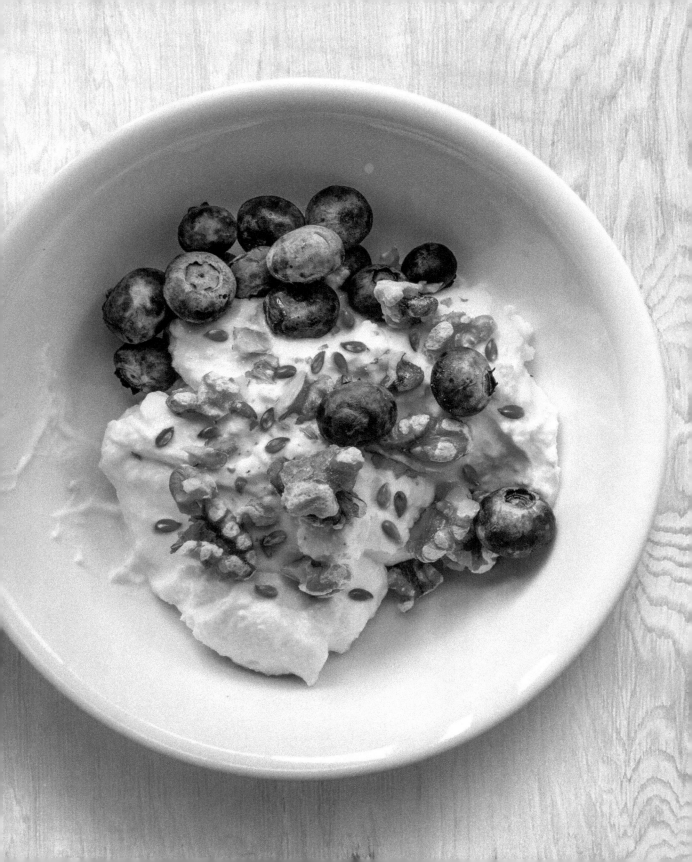

CHAPTER FOUR

Energizing
Breakfasts

Florentine Frittata

Serves 2   **PREP TIME:** 5 minutes | **COOK TIME:** 10 minutes

With detoxifying properties found in artichokes, herbs, and leafy greens, this healing frittata is one of my favorite go-to's for a quick and easy, yet filling and flavorful, breakfast. Look for free-range eggs, which are full of heart-healthy fatty acids, vitamins, and quality protein. A good alternative is cage-free or organic eggs. You can double this recipe and use a larger pan if you're feeding a crowd for brunch. And this frittata isn't just for breakfast! Leftover frittata is delicious over a mixed green salad with homemade vinaigrette for a light lunch.

4 eggs

¼ teaspoon salt

⅛ teaspoon freshly ground pepper

½ teaspoon dried or 1 tablespoon fresh chopped herbs such as rosemary, thyme, oregano, and basil (optional but adds flavor)

2 tablespoons olive oil

Handful fresh baby spinach or arugula leaves (about 1 cup)

8 cherry tomatoes, halved

4 ounces (½ cup) **canned quartered artichoke hearts, rinsed, drained, and thoroughly dried** (optional)

2 ounces soft goat cheese (optional, if including dairy)

1. Combine the eggs, salt, pepper, and herbs (if using) in a small bowl and whisk well with a fork. Set aside.

2. Preheat the broiler to 450°F and position a rack in the upper half of the oven.

3. Heat the oil in a small (4- to 5-inch) ovenproof skillet or omelet pan over medium heat. Add the spinach, tomatoes, and artichoke hearts and sauté 1 to 2 minutes, until the spinach is just wilted.

4. Pour in the egg mixture and let it cook undisturbed for 3 to 4 minutes over medium heat, or until the eggs begin to set on the bottom.

5. Breaking the goat cheese into clumps (if using), sprinkle along the top of the egg mixture and transfer the skillet to the oven.

6. Broil for another 3 to 4 minutes, or until the frittata is firm in the center and golden brown on top.

7. Remove the frittata from the oven and run a rubber spatula around the edge to loosen the sides. Transfer the frittata to a large plate or cutting board and slice it in half to make 2 servings. Serve warm or cold atop a salad for a light lunch.

SUBSTITUTION TIP You can substitute frozen spinach or other dark leafy greens for fresh, but make sure to reheat the frozen greens first and thoroughly drain all the liquid to avoid a soggy frittata.

PER SERVING Calories: 262; Total fat: 23g; Protein: 12g; Sodium: 429mg; Fiber: 1g

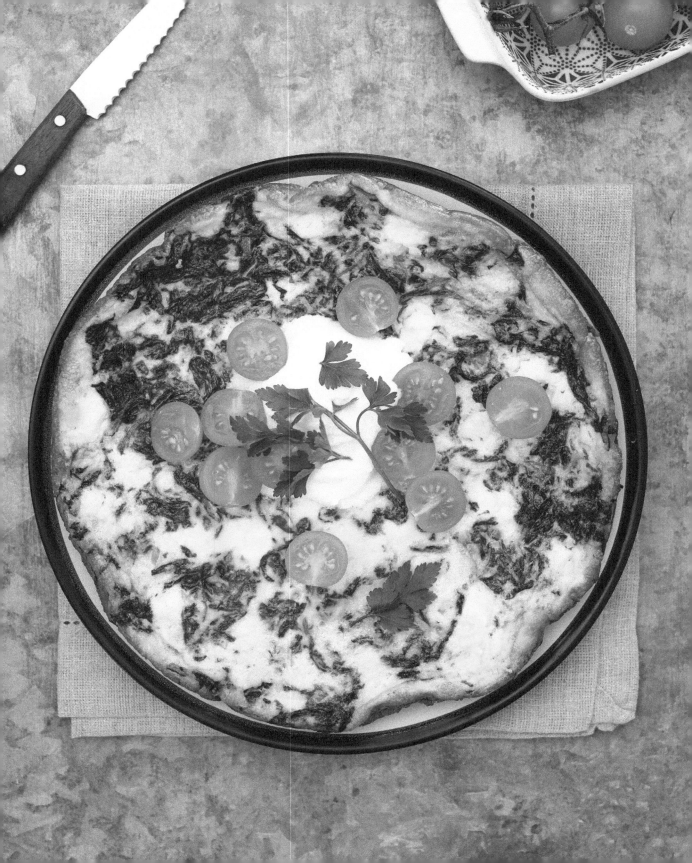

Yogurt Parfait

Serves 1   **PREP TIME:** 5 minutes

Quick and easy, this breakfast has it all: satiating heart-healthy fats, quality protein, probiotics, and antioxidants for cell and gut repair. You can use fresh berries in this parfait, but thawed frozen berries do a great job of naturally flavoring the plain yogurt with the juices they produce as they thaw.

½ **cup whole milk plain Greek yogurt** (preferably organic)

¼ **cup frozen blueberries, thawed with juices**

Dash vanilla or almond extract (optional)

Dash cinnamon (optional)

1 **tablespoon ground flaxseed**

2 **tablespoons chopped nuts** (walnuts or pecans work wonderfully)

1. Combine the yogurt, berries in their juice, extract (if using), cinnamon (if using), and flaxseed in a small bowl or glass. Stir well until smooth.

2. Stir in the nuts and enjoy.

PER SERVING Calories: 315; Total fat: 25g; Protein: 9g; Sodium: 53mg; Fiber: 5g

Avocado "Toast"

Serves 2   **PREP TIME:** 5 minutes | **COOK TIME:** 15 minutes

There's nothing better than the mix of textures from toast—crunchy on the outside and soft on the inside—topped with a creamy avocado. No need to say goodbye to this favorite combo just because bread is off-limits. This version of avocado "toast" satisfies the craving and is loaded with heart-healthy omega-3 fatty acids and protein. Top it with your favorite salsa (no sugar added) or hot sauce and some chopped fresh cilantro for a little kick.

2 eggs

2 tablespoons ground flaxseed

½ teaspoon baking powder

¼ teaspoon salt, plus more for seasoning

⅛ teaspoon freshly ground pepper, plus more for seasoning

¼ teaspoon garlic powder, sesame seed, caraway seed, or other dried herbs (optional)

1 tablespoon olive oil

1 medium avocado, pitted, peeled, and sliced

1. Combine the eggs, flaxseed, baking powder, salt, pepper, and herbs (if using) in a small bowl and whisk well, being sure to break up any clumps of ground flaxseed or baking powder. Let sit 2 minutes.

2. Heat the oil in a small nonstick skillet over medium heat. Pour the egg mixture into the skillet and let it cook undisturbed for 2 to 3 minutes, until the egg begins to set on the bottom.

3. Using a rubber spatula, scrape down the sides to allow the uncooked egg to reach the bottom. Repeat if needed (another 2 to 3 minutes).

4. Once almost set, flip like a pancake and allow the top to fully cook for another 1 to 2 minutes.

5. Remove from the pan and allow to cool slightly. Slice the cooked eggs into two pieces and toast them in a toaster oven until crisp.

6. Top the "toast" with the avocado slices and additional salt and pepper to taste.

PER SERVING Calories: 306; Total fat: 27g; Protein: 9g; Sodium: 653mg; Fiber: 8g

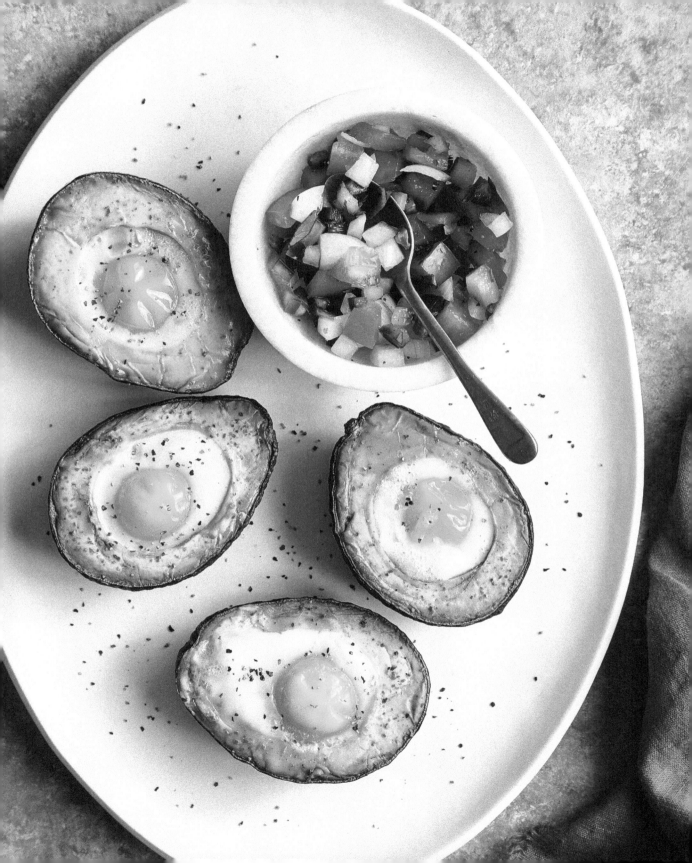

← Baked Egg in Avocado

Serves 2   **PREP TIME:** 2 minutes | **COOK TIME:** 15 minutes

Sure, scrambled eggs topped with avocado are a great breakfast staple, but sometimes I feel like I'm in a rut! This is a new spin on a classic favorite of mine, and you can really dress up this fun breakfast dish with the optional toppings. The baked avocados don't keep very well in the refrigerator, so make sure to prepare only what you're planning to eat in the moment.

1 large avocado, pitted and halved

2 eggs

Salt and pepper, to taste

OPTIONAL TOPPINGS

2 ounces cheese (optional, if including dairy)

Chopped fresh cilantro or basil, to taste

2 tablespoons salsa (no sugar added) **or** chopped tomatoes

2 ounces cooked and crumbled bacon or sausage

1. Preheat the oven to 425°F.
2. Scoop out 1 or 2 tablespoons from each avocado half to create a hole large enough to fit an egg. Place the avocado halves on a baking sheet, cut-side up.
3. Crack 1 egg into each avocado half and season with salt and pepper.
4. Bake until the eggs are set and cooked to your desired level of doneness (about 10 to 15 minutes).
5. Remove from the oven and top with optional ingredients, if using. If topping with cheese, return the avocados to the oven for another 2 to 3 minutes to melt the cheese.

PER SERVING Calories: 207; Total fat: 18g; Protein: 7g; Sodium: 146mg; Fiber: 6g

Southwestern Egg Muffins

Serves 6   **PREP TIME:** 5 minutes | **COOK TIME:** 25 minutes

I suggest making a batch of these muffins at the beginning of the two weeks and storing them in the freezer for a mid-week breakfast on the go. The cheese and sausage are optional. Feel free to mix up the spices for a different flavor, such as subbing rosemary and oregano for the cumin and chili powder and chopped basil for the cilantro to make a more Mediterranean version.

1 tablespoon olive oil, plus more for greasing the muffin tin

1 cup chopped bell pepper (orange, red, yellow, or green)

¼ cup chopped green onion

8 eggs

½ teaspoon ground cumin

½ teaspoon chili powder

½ teaspoon garlic powder

½ teaspoon salt

¼ teaspoon freshly ground pepper

½ cup chopped fresh cilantro (optional)

4 ounces cheese (optional, if including dairy)

4 ounces cooked and crumbled sausage (optional)

1 medium avocado, pitted, peeled, and chopped or ¾ cup guacamole, for serving

1. Preheat the oven to 350°F. Using a paper towel or your hands, grease the cups of a 12-count muffin tin with oil.

2. Heat 1 tablespoon oil in a medium skillet over medium heat. Sauté the peppers and green onions until tender and fragrant, about 2 to 3 minutes. Remove from the heat and allow to cool.

3. In a medium bowl, whisk the eggs, cumin, chili powder, garlic powder, salt, and pepper. Whisk in the pepper mixture, cilantro (if using), cheese (if using), and sausage (if using).

4. Divide the egg mixture evenly between the cups of the prepared muffin tin. Bake for 20 to 22 minutes, until the muffins are puffed up and cooked through.

5. Remove from the oven and allow to cool slightly. Serve warm with chopped avocado or guacamole.

STORAGE TIP Extra muffins can be cooled completely and stored in an airtight freezer bag for quick breakfasts throughout the next two weeks. Simply reheat in the microwave or oven before serving.

PER SERVING (2 muffins) Calories: 162; Total fat: 13g; Protein: 8g; Sodium: 282mg; Fiber: 3g

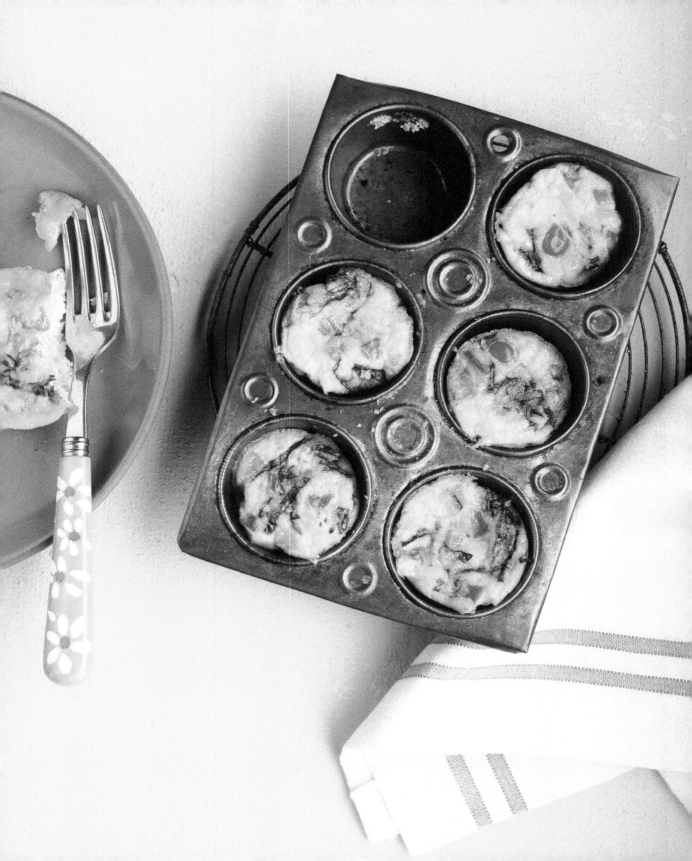

Grain-Free Pancakes with Berry Sauce

Serves 2   **PREP TIME:** 5 minutes | **COOK TIME:** 15 minutes

No need to give up weekend pancakes just because you are grain- and sugar-free! These pancakes are a delicious alternative to the original and are so tasty that the entire family will enjoy them. Use any frozen berry you like, but the pancakes are especially good with blueberries. If you are including dairy, you can whip up some organic heavy cream to dollop on top for a real treat.

FOR THE PANCAKES

½ cup almond flour

½ teaspoon cinnamon

½ teaspoon
  baking powder

3 tablespoons melted
  butter or coconut
  oil, divided

1 tablespoon water

¼ cup unsweetened
  almond or coconut milk

1 egg

½ teaspoon
  vanilla extract

1. Combine the dry ingredients (almond flour, cinnamon, and baking powder) in a medium bowl and whisk together to break up any clumps.
2. Add 2 tablespoons butter, the water, almond milk, egg, and vanilla, and whisk to combine.
3. Heat the remaining 1 tablespoon butter in a large skillet over medium heat and spoon in the batter to make 4 pancakes. Cook for 4 to 5 minutes, until bubbles begin to form, and flip to cook another 2 to 3 minutes on the second side.

FOR THE BERRY SYRUP

½ cup frozen berries

½ teaspoon
  vanilla extract

Juice of 1 clementine
(optional)

1. Heat the berries, vanilla, and clementine juice (if using) in a small saucepan over medium-high heat until bubbly, adding water if the mixture is too thick.
2. Using the back of a spoon or fork, mash the berries and whisk until smooth. Remove from the heat and serve over the pancakes.

PER SERVING Calories: 331; Total fat: 29g; Protein: 8g;
Sodium: 520mg; Fiber: 9g

Creamy Cauliflower "Oatmeal"

Serves 1   **PREP TIME:** 5 minutes | **COOK TIME:** 10 minutes

There's nothing quite like a warm and comforting bowl of oatmeal on a chilly morning. Just because you're grain-free doesn't mean you have to give up this indulgence. Amazingly enough, cauliflower makes a great oatmeal alternative, and with the addition of creamy almond butter and warm cinnamon, you may not even notice the difference. Add some of the optional stir-ins to change up the flavor and/or add extra healthy fat and protein. You can substitute other nut butters for the almond butter, but remember to avoid peanuts and peanut butter during the two-week program.

½ cup unsweetened almond or coconut milk

Dash vanilla or almond extract

½ teaspoon cinnamon

2 tablespoons unsweetened almond butter

1 cup riced cauliflower (see Preparation Tip)

Salt, to taste

OPTIONAL STIR-INS

1 or 2 tablespoons shredded unsweetened coconut flakes

1 tablespoon ground flaxseed

1 or 2 tablespoons chopped nuts

Fresh or frozen berries (limit to ¼ cup)

1. In a small saucepan over medium-high heat, whisk the together almond milk, vanilla, cinnamon, and almond butter. Bring to a boil, whisking occasionally.

2. Add the cauliflower and reduce the heat to medium-low for 8 to 10 minutes. Simmer until the cauliflower is cooked and the mixture has thickened.

3. Remove from the heat and add optional stir-ins for added flavor and nutrition.

PREPARATION TIP You can buy prepared riced cauliflower in the frozen vegetable section of most grocery stores. If you have a food processor, it is easy and more economical to make your own, freezing extra for later use. Simply core and remove any leaves or thick stalks from the head of one medium cauliflower and break it into florets. Add to a food processor and pulse until finely chopped or resembling the texture of rice.

PER SERVING Calories: 267; Total fat: 21g; Protein: 10g; Sodium: 367mg; Fiber: 8g

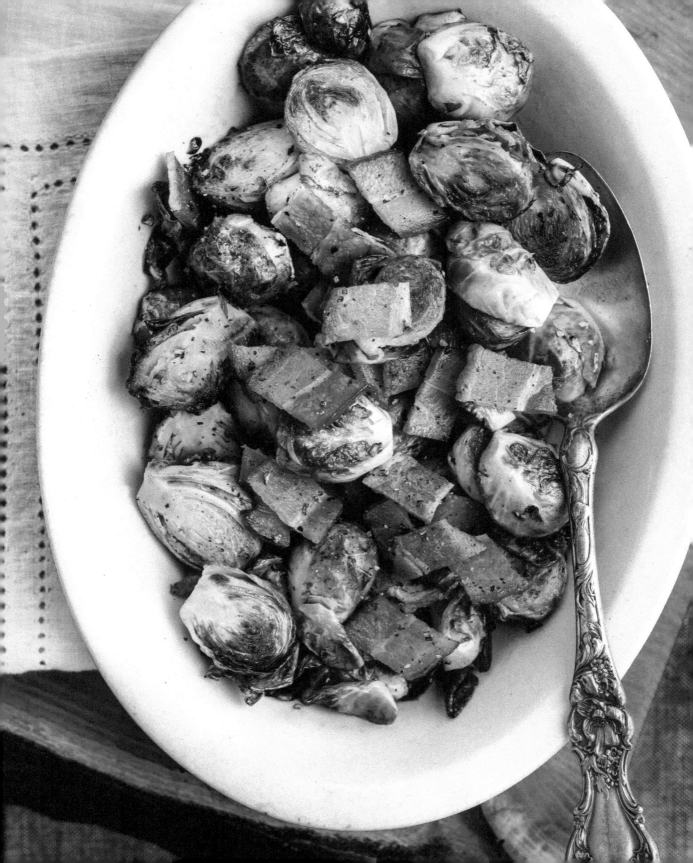

CHAPTER FIVE

Healthy
Lunches

Egg and Avocado Salad with Endive Spears

Serves 2   **PREP TIME:** 8 minutes | **COOK TIME:** 12 minutes + 1 hour to chill

Full of satiating protein and heart-healthy fats, this salad can be served with romaine hearts, celery spears, on its own, or over a bed of mixed greens. You can make a larger batch of this salad early in the week for a quick and easy portable lunch or light dinner. Feel free to mix up the fresh herbs for more variety: Basil, mint, and tarragon all work nicely!

4 eggs

1 medium avocado,
halved and pitted

1 tablespoon mayonnaise

1 tablespoon
Dijon mustard

Salt, to taste

Freshly ground pepper,
to taste

½ tsp dried or
2 tablespoons chopped
fresh dill (optional)

4 to 6 endive spears
(or romaine hearts)

1. Place the eggs in a medium saucepan and cover with room temperature water.

2. Set a timer for 12 minutes, place the saucepan over high heat, and bring the water to a boil. Reduce the heat to medium and gently boil the eggs until the 12 minutes is up.

3. Remove the eggs from the hot water and soak them in a small bowl of ice water for 3 to 4 minutes, until cool to the touch.

4. While the eggs cool, use a spoon to scoop out the insides of each avocado half and place the avocado in a medium bowl. Add mayonnaise, mustard, salt, and pepper, and dill (if using) and mash well with a fork until very creamy.

5. Once the eggs have cooled, peel them and chop them well. Add the eggs to the avocado mixture and stir to combine. Allow to chill in the fridge for at least 1 hour before serving.

6. Serve atop endive spears.

SUBSTITUTION TIP You can use canned or fresh cooked salmon, tuna, or shredded cooked chicken (see Tarragon Chicken Salad, page 91) instead of the chopped eggs, if desired.

PER SERVING Calories: 308; Total fat: 25g; Protein: 14g; Sodium: 354mg; Fiber: 9g

Healthy Fats Salad

Serves 1   **PREP TIME:** 10 minutes

I eat some version of this versatile salad almost daily! You can mix up the proteins, add or subtract ingredients based on what you have on hand, or prep everything in bulk to have a quick meal on busy days. Full of heart-healthy omega-3 fatty acids, quality proteins, and antioxidant-rich veggies, this easy salad is a winner!

FOR THE SALAD

2 to 4 cups greens, such as baby arugula, spinach, kale, or mixed salad

5 to 6 olives (green or black)**, pitted and roughly chopped**

1 small or ½ medium avocado, pitted, peeled, and sliced

1 or 2 tablespoons pumpkin seeds

3 or 4 ounces canned salmon, tuna (in oil)**, leftover chicken or other meat, or 2 hardboiled eggs**

Combine all the ingredients in a large bowl.

FOR THE DRESSING

2 tablespoons olive oil or avocado oil

2 tablespoons lemon juice (from 1 lemon) **or apple cider vinegar**

1 to 2 tablespoons freshly chopped herbs, such as basil, mint, oregano, or tarragon for added flavor (optional)

Salt, to taste

Freshly ground pepper, to taste

In a small bowl, whisk together the oil, lemon juice, herbs (if using), and season with salt and pepper. Drizzle the dressing over the salad and toss well to coat.

PER SERVING Calories: 605; Total fat: 57g; Protein: 16g; Sodium: 379mg; Fiber: 8g

Cream of Cauliflower Soup

Serves 2   **PREP TIME:** 10 minutes | **COOK TIME:** 25 minutes

Rich in flavor, a bowl of this soup is the perfect comfort food for a rainy day. As an added bonus, cauliflower contains sulforaphane, a phytochemical that assists in detoxification. This tasty soup is creamy enough on its own without any dairy and is the perfect guiltless indulgence that will help heal your body. Add cooked bacon, sausage, or shredded rotisserie chicken (see Tarragon Chicken Salad, page 91) for a heartier meal.

1 tablespoon olive oil

2 cups chopped cauliflower florets (about ½ a medium head) (can use frozen)

4 green onions, roughly chopped

2 garlic cloves, minced

1 cup water

2 tablespoons tamari

1 cup chopped kale

2 tablespoons chopped fresh basil

½ teaspoon salt

Chopped fresh parsley, to garnish (optional)

1. Heat the oil in a large soup pot over medium heat and sauté the cauliflower and green onions for 5 minutes until just golden. Add the garlic and sauté 1 minute more.

2. Add the water and tamari and bring to a boil. Reduce the heat to low and simmer, covered, for about 20 minutes or until the cauliflower is soft. Remove from the heat and allow the mixture to cool slightly.

3. Using an immersion blender (or stand blender, blending in batches), purée the mixture until smooth.

4. Add the kale, basil, and salt, and stir to combine. For a garnish, add parsley (if desired).

PER SERVING Calories: 127; Total fat: 7g; Protein: 6g; Sodium: 1,637mg; Fiber: 4g

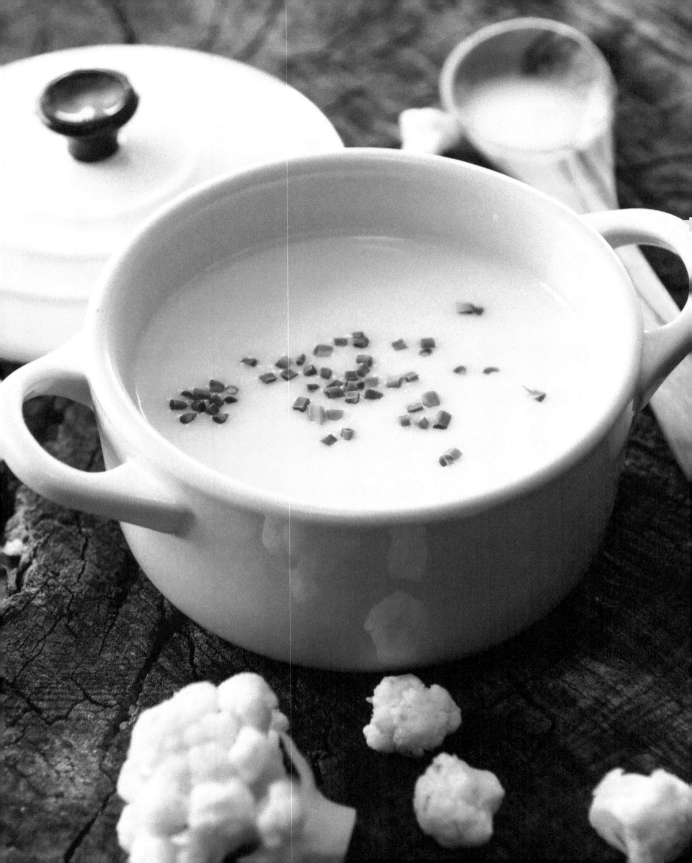

Roasted Eggplant Salad

Serves 2   **PREP TIME:** 10 minutes | **COOK TIME:** 30 minutes

Eggplant is rich in anthocyanin, the antioxidant responsible for its deep purple color, which helps protect cells (including those that line your GI tract) against damage. This salad is a great way to enjoy this often forgotten, nutrient-dense vegetable (that is technically a fruit!). I enjoy this salad both warm or chilled, depending on the season and my mood. For a stronger flavor, refrigerate the salad for at least an hour before serving. For a heartier meal, you can top each salad with a fried egg, 3 or 4 ounces of shredded cooked chicken (see Tarragon Chicken Salad, page 91), leftover cooked steak, or lamb.

FOR THE SALAD

1 **medium eggplant** (about 1 pound), **cut into ½-inch cubes**

4 **tablespoons olive oil**

1 **teaspoon salt**

¼ **teaspoon freshly ground pepper**

1 **small cucumber, peeled and diced**

1 **small bell pepper** (orange, red, or yellow), **seeded and chopped**

8 **to 10 cherry tomatoes, halved**

½ **cup chopped fresh mint leaves**

1. Preheat the oven to 400°F. Line a baking sheet with parchment paper and set aside.

2. Place the eggplant, oil, salt, and pepper in a large bowl and toss to coat well.

3. Place the eggplant on the prepared baking sheet and roast for 15 minutes, or until just beginning to soften. Reserve the large bowl for later use.

4. Remove the baking sheet from the oven and toss to flip the eggplant.

5. Return the baking sheet to the oven and roast until golden and cooked through for another 15 to 20 minutes.

6. Remove the baking sheet from the oven and transfer the cooked eggplant back to the large bowl.

7. Pour the dressing over the eggplant and toss to coat.

8. Add the cucumber, bell pepper, tomatoes, and mint and toss to combine.

9. Serve warm. Cover and refrigerate for up to 2 days.

FOR THE DRESSING

3 tablespoons fresh lime juice (about 2 limes)

1 tablespoon apple cider vinegar

¼ cup olive or avocado oil

Salt, to taste

Freshly ground pepper, to taste

Red pepper flakes, to taste (optional)

Whisk together the lime juice, vinegar, oil, salt, pepper, and red pepper flakes (if using) in a small bowl.

PER SERVING Calories: 560; Total fat: 51g; Protein: 5g; Sodium: 1,180mg; Fiber: 11g

Coleslaw Salad with Shredded Rotisserie Chicken

Serves 2   **PREP TIME:** 15 minutes + 1 hour to chill

Restaurant coleslaws are full of gut-disrupting added sugars, but with a delicious homemade alternative, you can include coleslaw in your backyard barbecues or this deliciously easy lunch salad recipe that incorporates store-bought rotisserie chicken. (For alternative ways to prepare the chicken, see Tarragon Chicken Salad, page 91.) Garnishing with a handful of fresh herbs is optional but adds a huge boost of anti-oxidants and amazing flavor. Mixing in more brightly colored veggies such as red cabbage, carrots, or even red bell peppers makes a very pretty presentation.

FOR THE COLESLAW DRESSING

1 tablespoon
  Dijon mustard

1 tablespoon apple
  cider vinegar

1 tablespoon fresh
  lemon juice

½ teaspoon salt

½ cup mayonnaise

¼ cup whole milk plain
  Greek yogurt

Freshly ground pepper,
  to taste

1. Combine the mustard, vinegar, lemon juice, salt, mayonnaise, yogurt, and pepper in a wide-mouthed mason jar or large bowl.

2. Whisk or blend with an immersion blender until smooth.

3. Cover, and refrigerate at least 1 hour before tossing with shredded cabbage or other raw veggies.

4. Extra dressing will last in the refrigerator for 1 to 2 weeks and is delicious with raw veggies or cooked meat or fish.

FOR THE SALAD

4 **cups shredded cabbage or bagged shredded coleslaw veggies** (any combination of red cabbage, green cabbage, carrots, broccoli, kale, etc.)

1 **cup cooked shredded chicken** (see Tarragon Chicken Salad, page 91)

1 **to 2 tablespoons fresh herbs, such as parsley, cilantro, or basil, to garnish** (optional)

1. Combine the shredded veggies with ½ cup of the dressing.

2. Add 1 cup cooked shredded chicken and the fresh herbs (if using) and toss well to coat. Divide the salad between two plates to serve.

PER SERVING Calories: 568; Total fat: 46g; Protein: 25g; Sodium: 1138mg; Fiber: 4g

Kale Salad with Lemon-Tahini Dressing

Serves 1 to 4   Dressing makes 1 cup   **PREP TIME:** 20 minutes

Commonly used in Middle Eastern, Greek, and Asian cuisines, tahini is a paste made from ground sesame seeds that gives hummus its creamy texture. Tahini is the backbone of many of my favorite dressings and sauces because it is so flavorful and packed with heart-healthy omega-3 fatty acids. It can be found jarred or canned in the ethnic foods or nut butter aisles of most grocery stores. Once opened, it can be stored in the refrigerator for several months. Make sure to stir the tahini well before using, because it separates easily.

FOR THE DRESSING

½ cup tahini

¼ cup fresh lemon juice (about 2 or 3 lemons)

¼ cup tamari (or liquid aminos)

1 tablespoon olive oil

1 garlic clove, pressed (or ½ teaspoon garlic powder)

1. Combine the tahini, lemon juice, tamari, oil, and garlic in a glass mason jar with a lid.
2. Cover and shake well until combined and creamy.
3. Store leftover dressing in a covered container in the fridge for up to 2 weeks.

FOR THE SALAD

2 to 4 cups fresh kale, de-ribbed, and torn into bite-size pieces

Place the kale in a large bowl and top with ¼ cup dressing. Toss to coat well and let sit for 15 minutes. The dressing will wilt the kale slightly to make it more tender. Toss the salad again before serving.

TIP You can top this salad with a protein of your choice such as leftover chicken or salmon or even a fried egg or two for a last-minute complete meal.

TIP Makes about 4 servings of dressing, which will store in the fridge for up to two weeks.

PER SERVING Calories: 24; Total fat: 10g; Protein: 4g; Sodium: 532mg; Fiber: 2g

Tarragon Chicken Salad

Serves 2   **PREP TIME:** 10 minutes

You can cook skinless chicken breasts or thighs either in a pressure cooker according to the manufacturer's instructions or in a pot of boiling water for about 20 to 25 minutes to have on hand for quick and easy mid-week meals. Alternatively, a store-bought rotisserie chicken makes for an easy option for precooked protein that can last for several meals.

¾ **cup** (6 ounces) **whole milk plain Greek yogurt**

1 **tablespoon Dijon mustard**

2 **tablespoons fresh lemon juice**

1 **teaspoon dried or 2 tablespoons chopped fresh tarragon**

Pinch garlic powder

Salt, to taste

Freshly ground pepper, to taste

1 **cup** (about 6 to 8 ounces) **cooked shredded chicken**

1. Combine the yogurt, mustard, lemon juice, tarragon, garlic powder, salt, and pepper in a medium bowl, and whisk until creamy.

2. Add the chicken and stir to coat.

TIP Serve this chicken salad with romaine or endive, topped on a mixed greens salad, or on its own with Seedy Crackers (page 109).

TIP Store leftover chicken salad in a covered container in the fridge for up to 4 days.

PER SERVING Calories: 6; Total fat: 3g; Protein: 27g; Sodium: 236mg; Fiber: 0g

Gut-Healing Chicken Soup

Serves 2   **PREP TIME:** 5 minutes | **COOK TIME:** 20 minutes

Collagen-rich bone broth is a great way to augment gut healing. Not everyone enjoys bone broth on its own, so here is a great way to incorporate it into your routine. This soup freezes very well, so you may want to double the batch and store some in the freezer for the coming weeks. You can add chopped celery or omit any of the chopped veggies if you don't have them on hand. But remember, the more color you add, the more antioxidants and cell-healing properties your soup will have!

2 tablespoons olive oil

½ cup chopped green onion

1 medium bell pepper (orange, red, or yellow), seeded and chopped

1 carrot, peeled and chopped

4 cups chicken bone broth

1 cup cooked shredded chicken (see Tarragon Chicken Salad, page 91)

1 or 2 cups fresh baby spinach, arugula, or kale leaves

Salt and pepper, to taste

¼ cup chopped fresh parsley (optional)

Red pepper flakes, to taste (optional)

1. Heat the oil in a medium saucepan over medium-high heat.
2. Add the green onion, bell pepper, and carrot, and sauté for 5 to 6 minutes, until tender.
3. Add the bone broth and bring to a boil. Add the chicken and greens.
4. Reduce the heat to low and simmer, covered, for 10 to 12 minutes or until the flavors develop, seasoning to taste with salt and pepper.
5. Serve with fresh parsley and red pepper flakes, if desired.

PER SERVING Calories: 36; Total fat: 16g; Protein: 42g; Sodium: 367mg; Fiber: 3g

Roasted Brussels Sprouts with Uncured Bacon

Serves 2   **PREP TIME:** 5 minutes | **COOK TIME:** 40 minutes

Even a Brussels sprouts hater will fall in love with this dish! Brussels sprouts are part of the family of cruciferous vegetables that is high in sulforaphane, making them wonderfully detoxifying. This dish is also delicious tossed with leftover Lemon-Tahini Dressing (see Kale Salad with Lemon-Tahini Dressing, page 90). For a heartier and higher-protein meal, top this dish with a fried egg or leftover cooked fish, chicken, or meat.

1 pound Brussels sprouts, halved

4 tablespoons olive oil

½ teaspoon salt

½ teaspoon garlic powder

¼ teaspoon freshly ground pepper

4 thick slices (about 2 ounces) **uncured bacon, cooked**

Lemon-Tahini Dressing (see page 90)**, for serving** (optional)

1. Preheat the oven to 425°F. Line a large baking sheet with parchment paper and set aside.

2. Place the Brussels sprouts in a large bowl. Sprinkle them with the oil, salt, garlic powder, and pepper, and toss well to coat.

3. Place the Brussels sprouts in a single layer on the prepared baking sheet and roast for 20 minutes. Set the large bowl aside for future use.

4. Remove the baking sheet from the oven and toss to flip the Brussels sprouts.

5. Return the baking sheet to the oven and continue to roast the Brussels sprouts for another 10 to 15 minutes, until browned and crispy.

6. Remove the baking sheet from the oven and return the Brussels sprouts to the large bowl. Add the bacon and Lemon-Tahini Dressing (if desired), and toss to combine well. Serve warm.

PER SERVING Calories: 397; Total fat: 30g; Protein: 12g; Sodium: 751mg; Fiber: 9g

Spiralized Veggie Salad

Serves 2   **PREP TIME:** 10 minutes | **COOK TIME:** 5 minutes

High in antioxidants and healthy fats, this salad makes a light vegetarian lunch. You can add cooked shredded chicken (see Tarragon Chicken Salad, page 91), canned salmon, or canned tuna to make this a heartier meal.

FOR THE SALAD

1 cup spiralized zucchini (1 zucchini)

1 cup spiralized carrot (from 1 carrot)

1 cup spiralized parsnip (from 1 or 2 parsnips)

5 or 6 radishes, cleaned and thinly sliced or shaved

½ cup fresh herbs (basil, cilantro, mint, or parsley)**, chopped**

Salt, to taste

Freshly ground pepper, to taste

1. Combine the zucchini, carrot, parsnip, radish, and the herbs in a large bowl.

2. While the dressing is still hot, pour it over the veggies and toss to coat. The hot dressing will tenderize the veggies slightly, but they will remain al dente.

3. Season with salt and pepper. Serve warm or chilled.

FOR THE DRESSING

2 tablespoons apple cider vinegar

2 tablespoons avocado or olive oil

2 tablespoons unsweetened almond butter

1. For the dressing, combine the vinegar, oil, and almond butter in a small saucepan over medium-high heat.

2. Whisking constantly, bring the mixture to a boil.

3. Turn off the heat and cover until ready to use.

PREPARATION TIP Already spiralized veggies can be found in the produce section of most grocery stores. You can easily make your own using a spiralizer (see "Kitchen Essentials," page 28).

PER SERVING Calories: 305; Total fat: 23g; Protein: 5g; Sodium: 58mg; Fiber: 7g

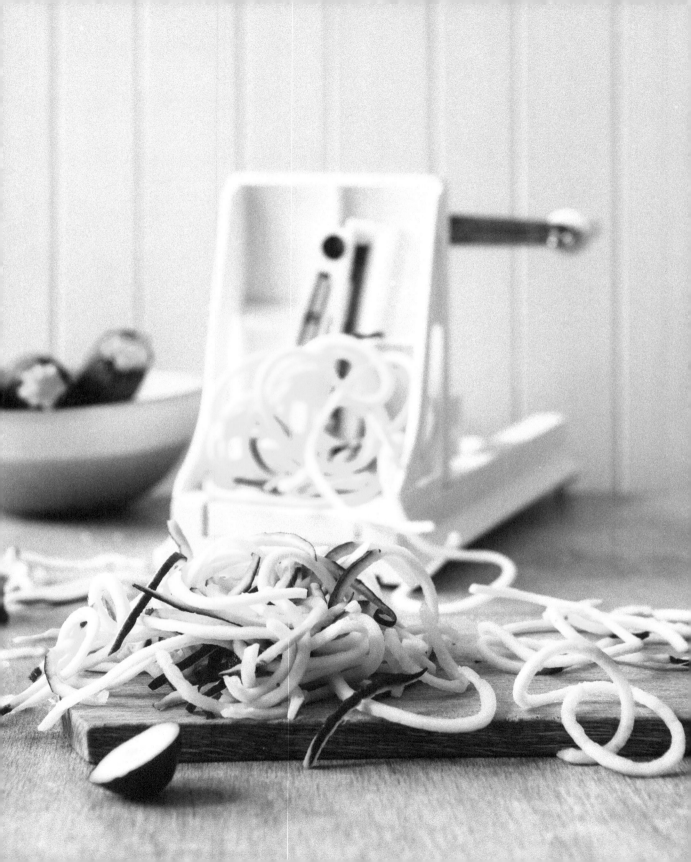

Creamy Lime-Cilantro Tuna Salad

Serves 1   **PREP TIME:** 10 minutes

This fresh take on an old classic makes canned tuna shine. With heart-healthy omega-3 fatty acids from the avocado and olive oil, this satiating salad is not only delicious but also packed with nutrition. I like using tuna packed in olive oil because it has a richer texture and more intense flavor. If using tuna packed in water, add an extra tablespoon of olive oil to the salad. Serve in lettuce wedges, atop a bed of mixed salad greens, or scoop it up by the spoonful on its own. It's that good!

FOR THE DRESSING

1 tablespoon water

¼ teaspoon salt

1½ teaspoons fresh lime juice

1 garlic clove

½ large ripe avocado, pitted and peeled

¼ cup packed fresh cilantro, leaves and stems coarsely chopped

1 tablespoon olive oil (add 1 tablespoon if using tuna packed in water)

Freshly ground pepper, to taste

Place the water, salt, lime juice, garlic, avocado, cilantro, olive oil, and pepper in a blender, and blend until thick and creamy.

FOR THE SALAD

4 ounces canned tuna, packed in olive oil, drained

1 to 2 cups greens, such as endive spears, romaine, or mixed salad greens, for serving

1. Combine the tuna with the dressing and serve with greens, if desired.

2. Extra dressing can be stored in the refrigerator for 2 to 3 days.

STORAGE TIP Avocado may turn brown after 1 or 2 days.

PER SERVING Calories: 485; Total fat: 37g; Protein: 32g; Sodium: 648mg; Fiber: 6g

Creamy Avocado Gazpacho

Serves 2   **PREP TIME:** 10 minutes

Full of heart-healthy omega-3 fatty acids from avocado, antifungal properties from apple cider vinegar, and probiotics from kefir, this is a powerhouse chilled soup. It doesn't freeze well and only stores in the fridge for a couple of days, so be sure to make only what you plan to eat within a week. You can add diced and seeded jalapeño if you like a little more heat.

2 or 3 pounds ripe tomatoes (preferably organic or heirloom)

1 medium bell pepper (orange, red, or yellow), **seeded and chopped**

¼ cup chopped fresh cilantro

¼ cup chopped green onion

1 medium cucumber, peeled and seeded (see Tip)

1 medium avocado, halved and pitted

3 tablespoons apple cider vinegar

Juice of 2 limes

1 tablespoon avocado oil

1 cup plain, whole milk kefir or Greek yogurt (preferably organic)

Salt, to taste

Freshly ground pepper, to taste

1. Combine the tomatoes, bell pepper, cilantro, onions, cucumber, avocado, vinegar, lime juice, oil, and kefir in a stand blender or wide cylindrical container. Using the stand blender or an immersion blender, blend everything until smooth and creamy.

2. Season to taste with salt and pepper and blend to combine the flavors.

3. Serve cold.

PREPARATION TIP To seed a cucumber, peel it first and then cut it in half widthwise. Quarter each half lengthwise and stand each quarter on its end. Take a knife down the length of the seeded side to remove the seeds.

PER SERVING Calories: 425; Total fat: 22g; Protein: 17g; Sodium: 79mg; Fiber: 16g

Thai Shrimp Spring Rolls

Serves 2   **PREP TIME:** 10 minutes | **COOK TIME:** 15 minutes

When you have a craving for take-out Asian food, this fits the bill. Full of flavor, it can also be served without lettuce wraps as a "fried rice" alternative. Feel free to mix up the protein if you don't eat shellfish: Fried egg, chicken, pork, or beef are great options.

2 tablespoons
coconut oil

1 medium carrot, peeled
and chopped

¼ cup chopped
green onion

8 ounces wild-caught
shrimp, peeled,
deveined, and cut into
bite-sized pieces

1 garlic clove, minced

1 cup riced cauliflower
(see Preparation Tip,
Creamy Cauliflower
"Oatmeal," page 79)

1 tablespoon fish sauce

1 tablespoon fresh lime
juice (from 1 small lime)

1 tablespoon sesame oil

¼ cup chopped fresh
mint (optional)

¼ cup chopped fresh
cilantro (optional)

Salt, to taste

Freshly ground pepper,
to taste

4 to 6 Bibb lettuce leaves

1 small avocado, pitted,
peeled, and sliced

1. Heat the oil in a large skillet over medium-high heat. Add the carrot and green onion and sauté for 5 to 6 minutes, until fragrant and just tender.

2. Add the shrimp and garlic and sauté for 4 to 5 minutes, until the shrimp just start to turn pink.

3. Add the cauliflower, fish sauce, lime juice, and sesame oil, and sauté for another 3 to 4 minutes, until the cauliflower is just tender.

4. Remove from the heat and stir in the mint and cilantro (if using) and season with salt and pepper.

5. Serve the shrimp and cauliflower mixture hot or cold in Bibb lettuce leaves with avocado slices, wrapping to create a spring roll shape.

PER SERVING Calories: 475; Total fat: 35g; Protein: 28g;
Sodium: 995mg; Fiber: 8g

Vietnamese Chopped Salad with Chicken

Serves 2   **PREP TIME:** 15 minutes

This light and refreshing salad is full of flavor. High in acetic acid, apple cider vinegar has the added benefit of being able to kill off many forms of bacteria, helping cleanse the gut and rebalance the microbiome. This is a complete meal with the addition of store-bought or leftover chicken, but you can substitute salmon if desired. Alternatively, as a vegetarian option, use scrambled eggs as your protein.

1 Thai chili, seeded and minced (optional for heat)

1 garlic clove, pressed or finely minced

2 tablespoons apple cider vinegar

2 tablespoons fresh lime juice (about 1 large or 2 small limes)

2 tablespoons Thai fish sauce (can substitute tamari but the fish sauce adds great flavor)

2 tablespoons sesame oil (can substitute olive oil or avocado oil)

¼ cup chopped green onion

1 small head Napa or Savoy cabbage, shredded or finely chopped

1 medium carrot, peeled and shredded

1 cup cooked shredded chicken (see Tarragon Chicken Salad, page 91)

½ cup chopped fresh mint or cilantro (or both)

1. Combine the chili, garlic, vinegar, lime juice, fish sauce, oil, and green onion in a large bowl and whisk well.

2. Add the cabbage, carrot, and chicken to the dressing and toss well.

3. Add the mint and/or basil and toss to combine. Serve at room temperature.

4. Extra salad will keep in the refrigerator for up to 4 days.

PER SERVING Calories: 288; Total fat: 16g; Protein: 25g; Sodium: 1,485mg; Fiber: 5g

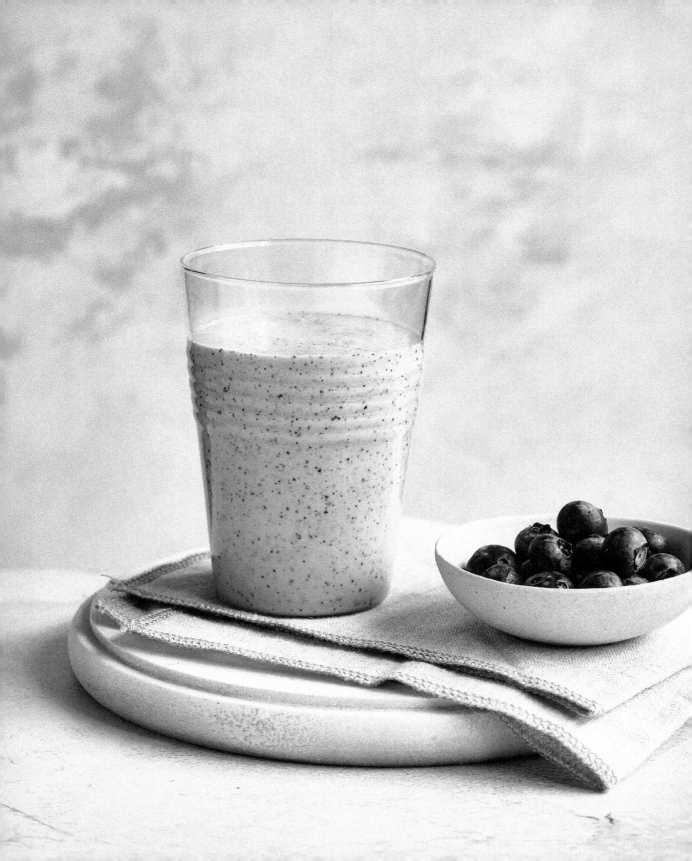

CHAPTER SIX

Savory Snacks
and Smoothies

Smoothies are a quick and convenient way to pack in a lot of nutrition on the go. For each smoothie recipe, simply combine all the ingredients in a blender (or wide-mouthed tall glass if using an immersion blender) and blend until smooth, adding additional ice or water to reach your desired thickness. Use organic dairy and produce, fresh or frozen, whenever possible. You can add extra protein as well as gut-healing power to any smoothie by adding a scoop of unflavored collagen peptides powder, available online or in health food stores.

Almond Joy Smoothie (Dairy-Free)

Serves 1   **PREP TIME:** 5 minutes

½ cup canned coconut milk

1 cup unsweetened almond milk

2 tablespoons unsweetened almond butter

1 tablespoon unsweetened cocoa powder

1 tablespoon unsweetened flaked coconut

Dash almond extract (to taste)

½ cup ice (optional)

Rich almond, coconut, and chocolate flavors come together in this delicious, satiating, and nutritious smoothie that makes a great breakfast or heartier snack for on-the-go days. Instead of using both the coconut and almond milks, you could opt to use only almond milk. This substitution would make the smoothie lighter and less creamy, but the full-fat canned coconut milk adds a rich and very satisfying texture—not to mention the added benefit of gut-healing properties and healthy fats.

PER SERVING Calories: 588; Total fat: 55g; Protein: 13g; Sodium: 182mg; Fiber: 11g

Probiotic-Rich Blueberry Smoothie

Serves 1   **PREP TIME:** 5 minutes

1 cup plain whole
  milk kefir

½ cup blueberries (fresh
  or frozen)

Juice of ½ lemon

Dash cinnamon, to taste

1 or 2 tablespoons
  ground flaxseed or chia
  seeds (optional)

Blueberries are high in antioxidants that help contribute to intestinal cell healing and support immune function. I like using frozen blueberries in smoothies because they add an icier texture, but you are welcome to use fresh if you have them. The base ingredient here, kefir, is an excellent source of lactose-free probiotics for restoring healthy gut balance.

PER SERVING Calories: 198; Total fat: 8g; Protein: 9g; Sodium: 130mg;
Fiber: 2g

Orange Creamsicle Smoothie

Serves 1   **PREP TIME:** 5 minutes

1 cup plain whole
  milk kefir

Juice of 2 clementines

Dash vanilla extract

Pinch cinnamon

1 to 2 tablespoons
  ground flaxseed or chia
  seeds (optional)

½ cup ice (optional)

Light and refreshing but full of gut-healing probiotic power, this smoothie is a great breakfast addition or midday snack. You can substitute the juice of 1 medium orange or tangerine for the clementine juice. Or, for another fun alternative, try topping with unsweetened coconut flakes for added flavor and crunch!

PER SERVING Calories: 191; Total fat: 8g; Protein: 9g; Sodium: 126mg; Fiber: 0g

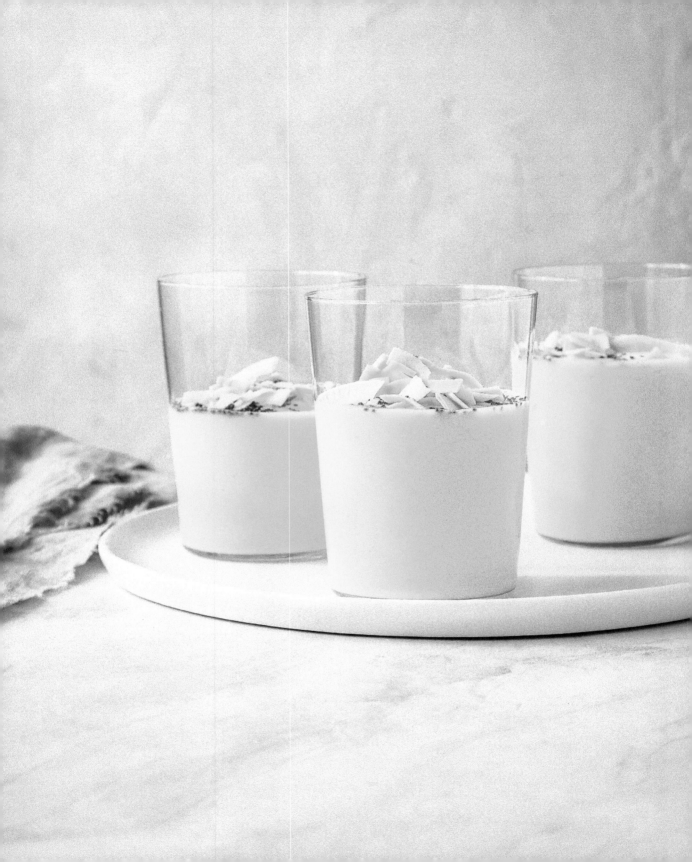

Gut-Healing Green Smoothie (Dairy-Free)

Serves 1 **PREP TIME:** 5 minutes

½ cup canned
    coconut milk

1 cup unsweetened
    almond milk

½ very ripe medium
    avocado, pitted
    and peeled

½ to 1 cup baby
    spinach leaves

Juice of 1 lime

¼ teaspoon
    powdered ginger

Pinch of cayenne pepper
    (optional)

½ cup ice (optional)

This is a dairy-free smoothie, but you can add ½ cup plain whole milk yogurt or kefir for probiotics if you're including dairy in your plan. High in heart-healthy omega-3 fatty acids from avocado and rich in vitamin C and calcium from spinach, this smoothie makes a powerhouse breakfast or light meal. It is also rich in fiber to help with digestive regularity.

PER SERVING Calories: 520; Total fat: 48g; Protein: 8g;
Sodium: 254mg; Fiber: 12g

Energy Balls

Makes about a dozen   **PREP TIME:** 20 minutes

These are the perfect on-the-go snack for busy days when you're out and about. With all-natural, whole-food ingredients rich in healthy fats and proteins, they will sustain you between meals. Everyone in my family loves these, and I send them in my kids' lunches daily. You'll never buy a processed granola or protein bar again!

1 cup unsweetened almond butter (all natural, no sugar added)

1 cup unsweetened coconut flakes

½ cup ground flaxseed meal

½ cup chopped nuts (walnuts or pecans work nicely)

¼ cup unsweetened cocoa powder

1 or 2 teaspoons pumpkin pie spice, cinnamon, or allspice (optional)

1. Combine all the ingredients in a large bowl.
2. Using your hands, mix everything together and shape the mixture into roughly a dozen 1-inch balls. Place them on a plate or cookie rack.
3. Store the balls in the refrigerator to chill and firm up before eating. They can also be kept in the freezer for up to 6 months.

PER SERVING (1 Energy Ball) Calories: 136; Total fat: 11g; Protein: 4g; Sodium: 43mg; Fiber: 5g

Chocolate and Almond Chia Pudding

Serves 2   **PREP TIME:** 10 minutes + 6 hours to chill

Chia seeds are high in omega-3 fatty acids as well as fiber for digestive health. This recipe makes a great snack or treat, so you may want to make a larger batch at the beginning of each week and store individual servings in smaller ramekins or glasses to have on hand during the workweek. You can change up the flavor by substituting ground ginger, allspice, pumpkin pie spice, or another favorite spice blend for the cinnamon, adding ¼ cup frozen berries in place of the almond butter and cocoa powder, or adding coconut flakes or chopped nuts for more texture. If you'd like, you could substitute more canned coconut milk for the almond milk to make the pudding richer and more satiating.

½ cup unsweetened almond milk

¼ cup canned coconut milk

¼ cup chia seeds

1 teaspoon cocoa powder

1 tablespoon almond butter

Pinch cinnamon, to taste

1. Combine all the ingredients in a small bowl, whisking well to incorporate the almond butter.
2. Divide the mixture between two ramekins, about ½ cup serving each.
3. Cover and refrigerate at least 6 hours, preferably overnight.
4. Serve cold.

PER SERVING Calories: 279; Total fat: 22g; Protein: 8g; Sodium: 100mg; Fiber: 12g

Seedy Crackers

Serves 2 to 4   **PREP TIME:** 20 minutes | **COOK TIME:** 15 minutes

These grain-free crackers are low in carbohydrates and high in healthy fats and protein to satisfy a craving for something crunchy without compromising your gut health. Enjoy them with Egg and Avocado Salad with Endive Spears (page 82), Tarragon Chicken Salad (page 91), a slice of avocado sprinkled with salt, or topped with smoked salmon. You can vary the ratios of seeds or increase the amount you use to suit your taste and preferred texture.

1 cup almond flour

1 tablespoon sesame seeds

1 tablespoon flaxseed

1 tablespoon chia seeds

¼ teaspoon baking soda

¼ teaspoon salt

½ teaspoon freshly ground pepper

1 egg (room temperature)

1. Preheat oven to 350°F.

2. Combine the almond flour, sesame seeds, flaxseed, chia seeds, baking soda, salt, and pepper in a large bowl and stir well.

3. In a small bowl, whisk the egg until well beaten.

4. Add the egg to the dry ingredients and stir well to combine, forming the dough into a ball.

5. Place a sheet of parchment paper on the countertop and place the dough on top. Cover with a second sheet of parchment and use a rolling pin to roll the dough out into a ⅛-inch thick rectangle.

6. Cut the dough into 1- to 2-inch crackers and bake on the parchment for 12 to 15 minutes, until crispy and slightly golden. Alternatively, you can bake the large rectangular dough sheet prior to cutting and break it into free-form crackers once baked and crispy.

7. Store the crackers in an airtight container in the fridge for up to 1 week.

PER SERVING Calories: 334; Total fat: 25g; Protein: 13g; Sodium: 496mg; Fiber: 8g

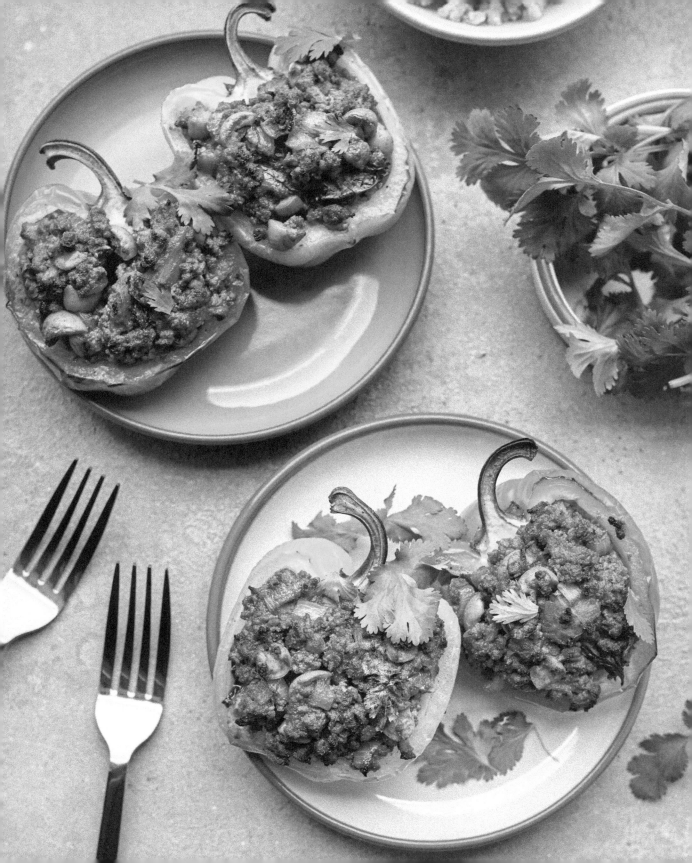

CHAPTER SEVEN

Delicious and Easy
Dinners

Spiced Meatballs in Coconut Curry over Cauliflower Rice

Serves 4   **PREP TIME: 15 minutes** | **COOK TIME: 40 minutes**

Dietitian fun facts: Cinnamon has been shown to have anti-inflammatory and some blood glucose-lowering effects when administered in conjunction with other treatment modalities, including diet and lifestyle. The cilantro is optional in this dish but adds wonderful anti-inflammatory micronutrients as well. This recipe freezes well, and I suggest that you freeze half to have on hand.

1 pound grass-fed ground beef

1 teaspoon cinnamon

1 teaspoon chili powder or paste (optional)

1 teaspoon garlic powder

1½ cups chopped cilantro, divided (optional)

3 tablespoons coconut oil, divided

4 garlic cloves, minced

2-inch piece of fresh ginger, peeled and minced

1 (13.5-ounce) **can coconut milk**

1 tablespoon curry powder (or red curry paste)

Juice and zest of 2 limes, divided

1. Place the ground beef, cinnamon, chili powder (if using), garlic powder, and ¾ cup of the cilantro in a large bowl, and combine well with a fork.

2. Using your hands, roll the mixture into 12 meatballs, about 1½ inches in diameter.

3. Heat 1 tablespoon of the coconut oil in a cast-iron skillet over medium-high heat.

4. Add the meatballs and brown them on all sides for 4 to 5 minutes.

5. Remove the meatballs from the skillet and keep warm, discarding all but 1 tablespoon of the drippings.

6. Reduce the heat to medium-low and scrape any browned bits of meat from the bottom of the skillet.

7. Add the minced garlic and ginger, and sauté 1 to 2 minutes.

8. Add the coconut milk, curry powder, and juice and zest of 1 lime, whisking to combine well.

9. Bring to a simmer and return the meatballs to the skillet. Reduce the heat to low, cover, and cook until the meatballs are heated through and the flavors develop, about 20 minutes.

10. While the meatballs cook, heat the remaining 2 tablespoons of coconut oil in a large skillet over medium-high heat.

4 cups finely riced cauliflower (see Preparation Tip, Creamy Cauliflower "Oatmeal," page 79)

Salt, to taste

Freshly ground pepper, to taste

11. Sauté the riced cauliflower for 4 to 5 minutes, stirring frequently, but making sure not to overcook the cauliflower.

12. Remove from the heat and toss with the juice and zest from 1 lime, the remaining ¾ cup cilantro, and salt and pepper to taste.

13. To serve, top 1 cup of the cauliflower with 3 meatballs and a fourth of the coconut curry sauce.

PER SERVING Calories: 552; Total fat: 44g; Protein: 28g; Sodium: 269mg; Fiber: 6g

Chicken Thighs with Creamy Arugula Pesto over Zucchini Noodles →

Serves 2   **PREP TIME:** 15 minutes | **COOK TIME:** 30 minutes

Arugula is chock-full of micronutrients (think vitamins and minerals). Both walnuts and olive oil are high in heart-healthy and anti-inflammatory omega-3 fatty acids.

2 cups arugula (packed)

1 cup fresh basil leaves

2 garlic cloves

½ cup chopped walnuts, toasted

½ cup shredded Parmesan cheese (not grated)

1 teaspoon salt, divided

½ teaspoon freshly ground pepper, divided

½ cup plus 1 tablespoon olive oil, divided

½ pound chicken thighs (2 [4-ounce] thighs or 4 smaller thighs)

1 tablespoon heavy whipping cream

4 cups spiralized zucchini noodles (about 2 large zucchinis; see Kitchen Essentials, page 28)

1. Combine the arugula, basil, garlic, walnuts, and cheese in a food processor and chop very finely. Add ½ teaspoon salt and ¼ teaspoon pepper.

2. With the processor running, pour in ½ cup oil until well blended. If the mixture seems too thick, add warm water 1 tablespoon at a time until the texture is smooth and creamy.

3. Heat the remaining 1 tablespoon of oil in a large skillet over medium-high heat.

4. Season the chicken thighs with the remaining ½ teaspoon salt and ¼ teaspoon pepper.

5. Add the chicken to the hot skillet and brown for 3 to 4 minutes on each side.

6. Remove the thighs from the skillet and cover to keep warm.

7. Reduce the heat to low, add the arugula pesto and cream, and whisk to combine.

8. Bring to a simmer, add the chicken thighs back to the skillet, reduce the heat to low, and cover. Cook for another 15 to 20 minutes, until chicken is heated through.

9. Serve 1 chicken thigh over raw spiralized zucchini "zoodles," spooning the sauce over top to cover.

TIP Make additional pesto to freeze for later or mix with shredded cooked chicken (see Tarragon Chicken Salad, page 91) for an easy chicken salad or with scrambled eggs for an easy weekday breakfast.

PER SERVING Calories: 579; Total fat: 5g; Protein: 19g; Sodium: 486mg; Fiber: 3g

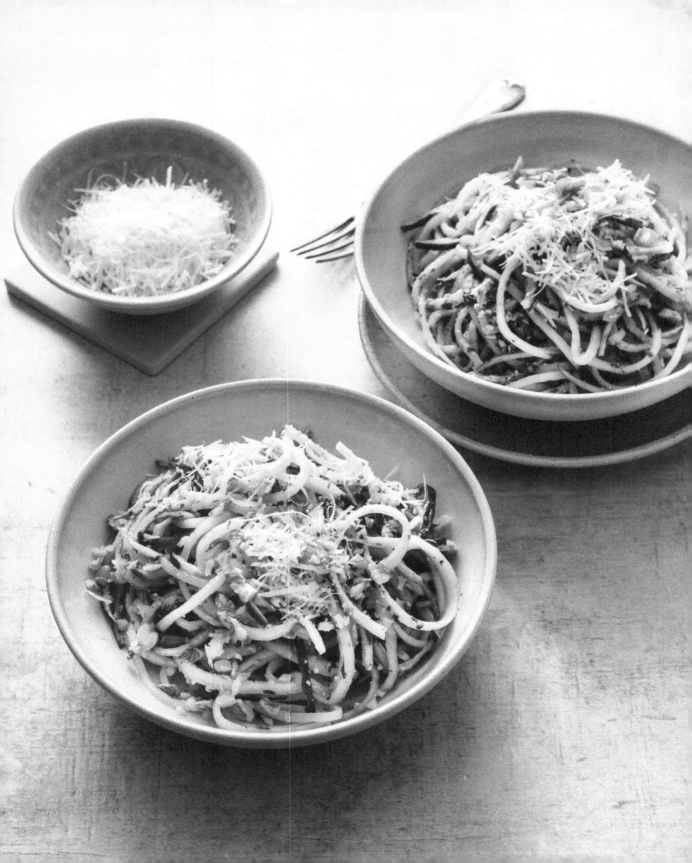

Slow Cooker Greek Chicken with Cauliflower Tabouli

Serves 4   **PREP TIME:** 15 minutes | **COOK TIME:** 6 hours

Slow cookers (Crock-Pots or Instant Pots®) are huge time-savers that create dishes with complex flavors. The variety of herbs in this tabouli adds so much flavor, as well as phytochemicals for improved immunity and cell repair. Any leftover chicken is great over a mixed greens salad for a quick and easy lunch.

FOR THE CHICKEN

1 pound boneless, skinless chicken thighs (preferably organic)

2 lemons, thinly sliced (with peel)

6 garlic cloves, smashed with the back of a knife

1 teaspoon dried dill (optional)

1 teaspoon dried oregano (optional)

½ teaspoon salt

½ teaspoon freshly ground pepper

2 tablespoons olive oil

1 cup chicken stock (or water)

1. Place the chicken, lemons, garlic, dill (if using), oregano (if using), salt, and pepper in a slow cooker and stir to coat well.

2. Pour the oil and stock over the chicken to cover it, adding additional liquid if needed.

3. Cook on low heat for 6 hours, or according to manufacturer's instructions.

4. Once the chicken has finished cooking, remove the lemons from the slow cooker and discard.

5. Using two forks, shred the chicken and serve with the broth from the slow cooker and 1 cup of cauliflower tabouli.

6. You can freeze half of this recipe, if desired.

FOR THE TABOULI

3 tablespoons olive
  oil, divided

4 cups riced cauliflower
  (from 1 medium head
  cauliflower; see
  Preparation Tip, Creamy
  Cauliflower "Oatmeal,"
  page 79)

1 cucumber, peeled,
  seeded, and chopped

¼ cup quartered cherry
  tomatoes

1 cup baby arugula leaves

¼ cup chopped
  mint leaves

¼ cup chopped Italian
  parsley

Juice of 1 lemon

1 garlic clove, pressed or
  finely minced

Salt, to taste

Freshly ground pepper,
  to taste

1. For the tabouli, heat 1 tablespoon oil in a large skillet over medium-high heat. Sauté the riced cauliflower for 5 to 8 minutes, until just tender but not mushy.

2. Transfer the cauliflower to a large bowl. Allow it to cool slightly.

3. Add the cucumber, tomatoes, arugula, mint, and parsley, and stir to combine.

4. In a small bowl, whisk together the remaining 2 tablespoons olive oil, lemon juice, and garlic.

5. Pour the dressing over the cauliflower and toss to coat. Season to taste with salt and pepper and serve slightly warm or at room temperature.

PER SERVING Calories 353; Total fat: 2Servingg; Protein: 26g;
Sodium: 435mg; Fiber: 6g

Salmon Cakes with Asparagus Almondine

Serves 4   **PREP TIME:** 20 minutes + 15 minutes resting | **COOK TIME:** 25 minutes

Salmon is packed with heart-healthy and anti-inflammatory omega-3 fatty acids. You can use fresh skinless fillets, but canned salmon typically contains tiny bones that are softened by the canning process and not detectable in the final product, adding calcium.

1 (14.5-ounce) **salmon fillet, skin removed** (sockeye is preferred) **or 1** (1-pound) **wild-caught salmon fillet, skin removed**

1 egg

2 tablespoons mayonnaise

1 medium very ripe avocado, well mashed

½ cup almond flour

½ cup minced red onion

1 teaspoon garlic powder

1 teaspoon dried dill

2 teaspoons Old Bay seasoning (preferably low sodium)

4 tablespoons olive oil, divided

4 garlic cloves, minced

4 cups (about 1 pound) **asparagus spears, rough ends trimmed**

Salt, to taste

Freshly ground pepper, to taste

½ cup slivered almonds, lightly toasted

1. Place the salmon in a large bowl and use a fork to break the fillet up into small pieces. Add the egg, mayonnaise, avocado, almond flour, onion, garlic powder, dill, and Old Bay seasoning, and combine well.

2. Form into 8 small patties, about 2 inches in diameter. Let sit for 15 minutes.

3. Heat 2 tablespoons oil in large cast-iron skillet over medium heat.

4. Fry the patties for 2 to 3 minutes per side until browned.

5. Cover the skillet, reduce the heat to low, and cook another 6 to 8 minutes, or until the patties are set in the center.

6. Remove the patties from the skillet and cover to keep warm.

7. Heat the remaining 2 tablespoons oil in the same skillet over medium heat.

8. Add the garlic, asparagus, salt, and pepper, and sauté for 6 to 8 minutes, until just barely tender, being sure not to overcook the asparagus or burn the garlic.

9. Remove the asparagus from the skillet and top with the almonds. Serve warm.

TIP Almonds, almond flour, and avocado are high not only in omega-3 fatty acids but also fiber, which helps with constipation—a common side effect when cutting back on whole-grain carbohydrates. These salmon cakes are very freezer-friendly and make a convenient mid-week lunch atop a salad.

PER SERVING Calories: 601; Total fat: 46g; Protein: 32g; Sodium: 454mg; Fiber: 9g

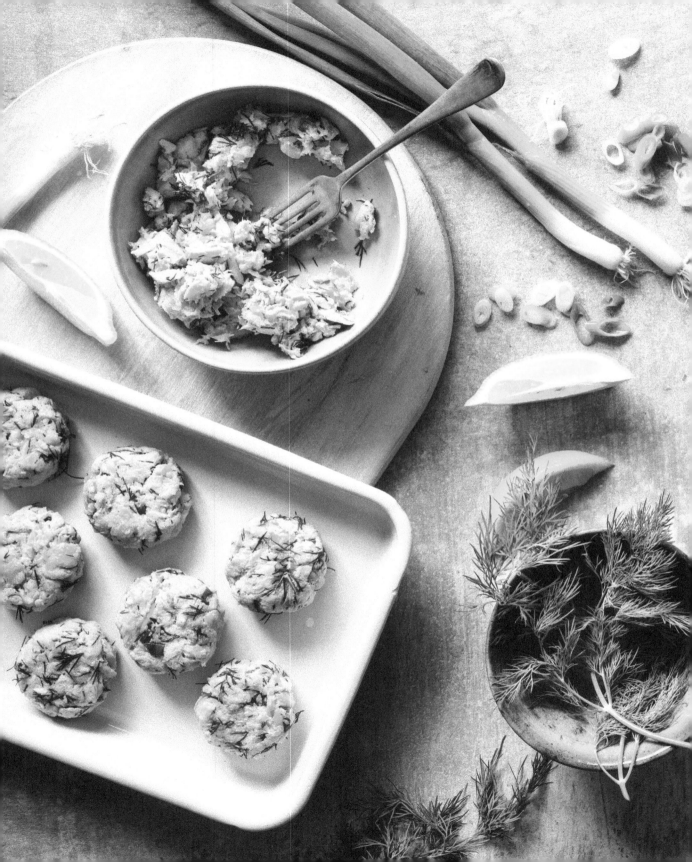

Southwestern Stuffed Peppers

Serves 2   **PREP TIME:** 10 minutes | **COOK TIME:** 35 minutes

Loaded with anti-inflammatory antioxidants from the colorful peppers, this is a quick and easy weeknight meal that also freezes well. You can substitute ground turkey or chicken for the beef if you prefer. If you are including dairy, you can top each pepper with a small handful of shredded cheese just before baking. I love to eat these cold the next day for a quick lunch—just like leftover cold pizza!

2 bell peppers (orange, red, or yellow)**, halved and seeded**

2 tablespoons olive oil, divided

½ teaspoon salt

¼ teaspoon freshly ground pepper

4 green onions, thinly sliced

2 garlic cloves, minced

½ pound ground beef (preferably grass-fed)

1 teaspoon chili powder

1 teaspoon ground cumin

½ teaspoon paprika

Pinch cayenne pepper (optional, for spice)

½ cup (4 ounces) **canned diced tomatoes**

¼ to ½ cup chopped cilantro (optional)

2 limes wedges (for serving)

1. Preheat oven to 400°F.
2. Arrange the pepper halves on a baking sheet and drizzle with 1 tablespoon oil. Sprinkle with salt and pepper and bake for 8 to 10 minutes, until softened.
3. Heat the remaining 1 tablespoon oil in a large skillet over medium-high heat.
4. Add the green onions and garlic and cook for 4 to 5 minutes, until softened.
5. Add the ground beef, breaking it up as it browns, and cook for 4 to 5 minutes.
6. Stir in the chili powder, cumin, paprika, and cayenne pepper (if using) and cook for an additional 30 seconds.
7. Add the tomatoes and let simmer for 5 minutes, uncovered.
8. Stir in the cilantro (if using) and mix well.
9. Fill the softened peppers with the beef mixture and bake for 10 minutes.
10. Serve with lime wedges.

PER SERVING Calories 388; Total fat: 26Serving; Protein: 27g; Sodium: 951mg; Fiber: 4g

Sage and Citrus Roasted Pork Chops

Serves 2   **PREP TIME:** 5 minutes | **COOK TIME:** 30 minutes

You can use boneless chops in this recipe, but bone-in yields a moister pork chop with deeper flavor. Double the recipe to have leftovers for lunches throughout the week. These are great with a simple salad or sautéed kale or spinach.

2 bone-in thick-cut pork chops (about 1 pound, or 8 ounces if using boneless chops)

4 to 6 fresh sage leaves, chopped (or 1 teaspoon dried sage)

2 garlic cloves, smashed with the back of a knife

1 lemon, thinly sliced (with peel)

1 orange or tangerine, thinly sliced (with peel)

2 tablespoons olive oil

½ teaspoon salt

¼ teaspoon freshly ground pepper

1. Preheat the oven to 450°F.
2. Place the pork chops in a medium glass baking dish just large enough to fit the chops.
3. In a small bowl, combine the sage, garlic, lemon slices, orange slices, and oil. Using the back of a spoon, squeeze some juice from the lemon and orange, and stir well to combine.
4. Pour the citrus mixture over the pork, season with salt and pepper, and turn to coat.
5. Cover the pork with foil or a glass lid and roast until the pork is cooked through, 25 to 30 minutes for bone-in and 20 to 25 minutes for boneless, depending on the thickness of the chops.

PER SERVING Calories: 355; Total fat: 25g; Protein: 22g; Sodium: 434mg; Fiber: 3g

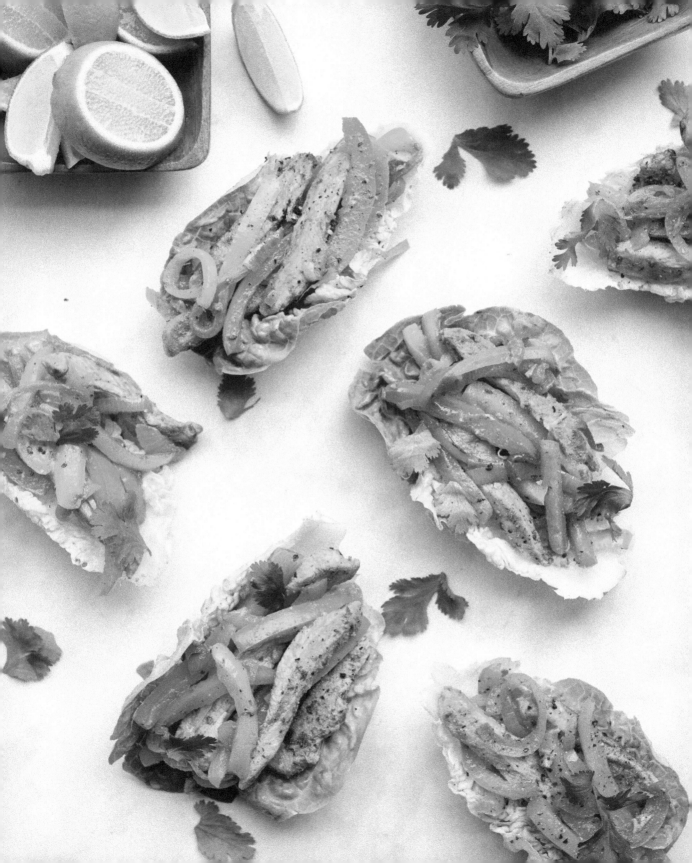

← Fajita Bowl and Wraps

Serves 2 | **PREP TIME:** 10 minutes | **COOK TIME:** 10 minutes

Leftover Cumin-Spiced Flank Steak (page 125), Slow Cooker Pork Carnitas (page 129), or store-bought rotisserie chicken make this dish come together in a flash.

1 tablespoon olive oil

1 bell pepper (orange, red, or yellow)**, seeded and sliced**

4 green onions, chopped

1 garlic clove, minced

8 ounces leftover Cumin-Spiced Flank Steak (page 125), Slow Cooker Pork Carnitas (page 129)**, or chicken** (organic)

½ teaspoon chili powder blend (optional)

Salt, to taste

Freshly ground pepper, to taste

2 to 4 cups greens, such as baby spinach, arugula, or kale

1 medium avocado, pitted, peeled, and sliced

OPTIONAL GARNISHES

2 lime wedges

1 to 2 tablespoons chopped cilantro

1 to 2 tablespoons plain whole milk Greek yogurt

1 to 2 tablespoons salsa, no sugar added

1 to 2 tablespoons chopped tomato

1. Heat 1 tablespoon olive oil in a large skillet over medium-high heat.

2. Sauté the bell pepper and green onions for 5 minutes. Add the minced garlic and sauté for another 2 to 3 minutes, or until the peppers are tender.

3. Add the meat, chili powder (if using), salt, and pepper, and toss to coat. Sauté for another 2 to 3 minutes, or until the flavors are well blended.

4. Divide the greens between two bowls and top each with half the meat and pepper mixture. Top with sliced avocado and any of the optional garnishes (lime, cilantro, yogurt, salsa, or tomato). Enjoy warm.

FUN TIP Instead of using a bowl, try scooping this dish into lettuce leaves to make a healthy and fun wrap.

PER SERVING Calories: 364; Total fat: 24g; Protein: 30g; Sodium: 198mg; Fiber: 9g

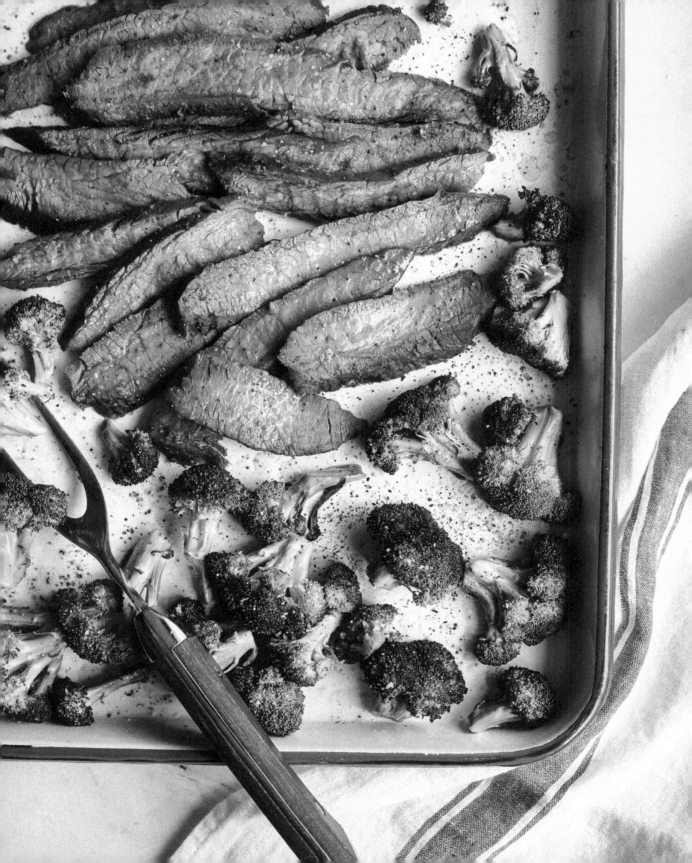

← Cumin-Spiced Flank Steak with Roasted Broccoli

Serves 2 (with leftover steak)   **PREP TIME:** 20 minutes | **COOK TIME:** 30 minutes

Use leftover steak atop a salad for lunch or in the Fajita Bowl and Wraps recipe (page 123). You can roast any vegetable to accompany the steak: Cauliflower, asparagus, green beans, and eggplant are all great. The key is making the veggie pieces a uniform size and adding enough oil to prevent burning. You can add variety with various spices and herbs to fit your palate.

5 tablespoons olive oil, divided

2 teaspoons ground cumin

1 teaspoon chili powder

1½ teaspoons garlic powder, divided

1½ teaspoons salt, divided

1 to 1½ pounds flank steak

2 cups broccoli florets

¼ teaspoon freshly ground pepper

1. Preheat the oven to 425°F and heat a grill to medium heat.

2. Combine 1 tablespoon oil, the cumin, chili powder, 1 teaspoon garlic powder, and 1 teaspoon salt in a small bowl to form a paste.

3. Rub the steak with the seasoning and let it sit for 15 minutes.

4. Place the broccoli, remaining 4 tablespoons of oil, remaining ½ teaspoon of salt, remaining ½ teaspoon of garlic powder, and pepper in a large bowl, and toss to coat well.

5. Spread out the broccoli in a single layer on a rimmed baking sheet and bake 20 to 25 minutes, until browned and slightly tender, tossing to flip halfway through the cooking time.

6. Place the steak on the grill and cook 6 to 9 minutes per side, or to your desired doneness.

7. Remove the steak from the grill and allow it to rest 5 minutes before slicing.

8. Serve while the steak and broccoli are warm.

9. Leftover steak will keep in the fridge for 4 to 5 days.

PER SERVING Calories: 682; Total fat: 49g; Protein: 53g; Sodium: 1,792mg; Fiber: 3g

Stir-Fried Beef and Broccoli

Serves 1 to 2   **PREP TIME:** 10 minutes + 30 minutes to marinate | **COOK TIME:** 20 minutes

Most store-bought stir-fry sauces are chock-full of sugars! Luckily, it's easy to make your own, and with enough flavor, you won't miss the sugar and high-fructose corn syrup. Your gut will thank you!

1-inch piece of fresh ginger, peeled and roughly chopped

1 garlic clove

2 tablespoons chopped green onion

Red pepper flakes, to taste (optional)

2 tablespoons water

2 tablespoons tamari

1 tablespoon sesame oil (can substitute with avocado oil for a less intense flavor)

1 (8-ounce) **flank steak, sliced**

2 tablespoons olive oil, divided

2 cups broccoli florets

1. To make the marinade, combine the ginger, garlic, green onion, red pepper flakes (if using), water, tamari, and sesame oil in a blender and purée until the ginger is finely minced.

2. Place the marinade in a glass bowl and add the sliced flank steak. Cover and refrigerate at least 30 minutes (or overnight).

3. Heat 1 tablespoon olive oil in a large skillet over medium-high heat. Remove the steak from the marinade and add it to the skillet, reserving the marinade liquid.

4. Stir-fry the steak in oil for 4 to 5 minutes, until browned on all sides. Remove from the skillet and keep warm.

5. Add the remaining 1 tablespoon oil to the skillet, reduce the heat to medium, and stir-fry the broccoli for 4 to 5 minutes, until slightly browned. Return the steak to the skillet, add the reserved marinade, and stir to combine.

6. Cover and cook over medium-low heat until the meat is cooked through and the broccoli is tender, about 10 minutes.

PREPARATION TIP For a more intense flavor, you can double the amount of ginger and garlic in the sauce.

PER SERVING Calories: 844; Total fat: 62g; Protein: 59g; Sodium: 2,073mg; Fiber: 5g

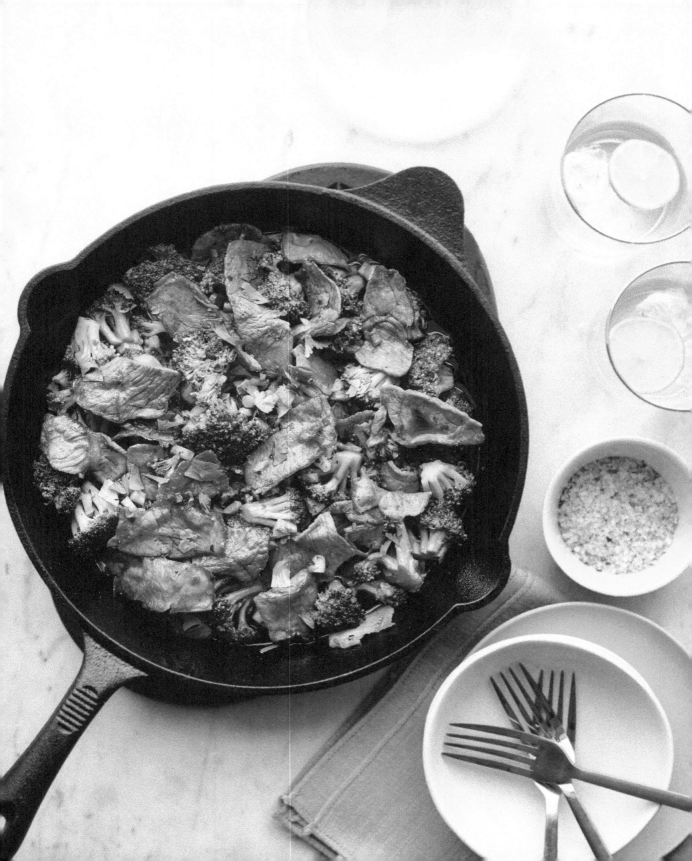

Crispy Coconut Salmon

Serves 2   **PREP TIME:** 20 minutes | **COOK TIME:** 20 minutes

Crispy on the outside and moist on the inside, this salmon has a wonderful texture and flavor. You can substitute almond flour for the coconut flour in this recipe, if desired. Serve over a bed of greens with a light vinaigrette or with roasted or stir-fried asparagus or broccoli.

2 tablespoons melted coconut oil, divided

¼ cup coconut flour

½ cup unsweetened flaked coconut

½ teaspoon salt

¼ teaspoon freshly ground pepper

1 egg

1 (8-ounce) **skinless salmon fillet, cut into 2 pieces**

2 teaspoons stone-ground mustard

2 lime wedges, for serving (optional)

1. Preheat the oven to 375°F.
2. Brush a baking sheet with 1 tablespoon melted coconut oil and set aside.
3. In a small bowl, combine the coconut flour, shredded coconut, salt, and pepper.
4. In a separate small bowl, beat the egg.
5. Dip one salmon fillet into the egg, coating both sides evenly. Transfer the fillet to the coconut mixture and coat both sides evenly. Place the salmon onto the prepared baking sheet. Repeat with the other salmon fillet. Drizzle both with the remaining 1 tablespoon melted coconut oil.
6. Bake the salmon for 15 to 18 minutes, or until the fish is tender and the coconut crust is golden brown. Serve with stone-ground mustard and lime wedges, if desired.

PER SERVING Calories: 525; Total fat: 41g; Protein: 25g; Sodium: 667mg; Fiber: 9g

Slow Cooker Pork Carnitas

Serves 6 to 8   **PREP TIME:** 10 minutes | **COOK TIME:** 8 hours and 30 minutes

This recipe makes a lot of pork. I suggest freezing half of this recipe for later use and thawing it to use as a topping for mid-week salads, as an addition to scrambled eggs, or in the Fajita Bowl and Wraps recipe (page 123). This dish is a flavorful, mostly hands-off crowd-pleaser. Serve with a side of coleslaw (see Coleslaw Salad with Shredded Rotisserie Chicken, page 88) for a complete meal.

2 tablespoons olive oil

2 or 3 pounds boneless pork loin, cut into 4 or 6 large chunks

6 garlic cloves, smashed with the back of a knife

2 teaspoons ground cumin

1 teaspoon chili powder

½ teaspoon ground cinnamon

½ teaspoon dried oregano

1 or 2 tablespoons chopped chipotle chili peppers in adobo sauce (optional)

1 teaspoon salt

¼ teaspoon freshly ground pepper

1 to 2 cups chicken broth

OPTIONAL GARNISH FOR SERVING

1 cup sliced radish

6 to 8 lime wedges

2 large avocados, pitted, peeled, and sliced

1 cup chopped cilantro

1. Heat the oil in a slow cooker turned to high heat. (For an Instant Pot®, use the sauté mode.)

2. Place the pork in the heated oil. Add the garlic and cumin, chili powder, cinnamon, oregano, chili peppers, salt, and freshly ground pepper, and stir to coat the meat.

3. Brown the pork on all sides, turning every 2 to 3 minutes. Once browned, reduce the heat to low and cover with chicken broth.

4. Set the timer for 6 to 8 hours.

5. After the time is up, use 2 forks to shred the cooked pork and return the slow cooker to high heat. Sauté 15 to 20 minutes, uncovered, or until the liquid has reduced by half and the pork is slightly crispy.

PER SERVING Calories: 256; Total fat: 12g; Protein: 33g; Sodium: 601mg; Fiber: 1g

Creamy Lemon Tarragon Baked Salmon

Serves 2   **PREP TIME:** 10 minutes | **COOK TIME:** 15 minutes

This is my go-to salmon recipe because it's easy enough for a weeknight but fancy enough for entertaining. This light and creamy dish will convert even a non-salmon lover to the heart-healthy protein! You can substitute another dried herb such as basil, oregano, or rosemary for the tarragon, if desired. The sauce in this recipe is also a wonderful base for chicken salad.

2 tablespoons high quality mayonnaise (such as avocado)

2 tablespoons Dijon or stone-ground mustard

Juice and zest of ½ lemon

1 teaspoon dried tarragon

½ teaspoon salt

¼ teaspoon freshly ground pepper

1 (8- to 10-ounce) **salmon fillet** (skin on is fine)

1. Preheat the oven to 375°F.
2. In a small bowl, whisk together the mayonnaise, mustard, lemon juice and zest, tarragon, salt, and pepper.
3. Place the salmon fillet, skin-side down, on a baking sheet lined with parchment paper.
4. Top the salmon with the sauce mixture, spreading evenly.
5. Bake 8 to 15 minutes, or until the salmon is slightly browned and cooked to your desired degree of tenderness.

PER SERVING   Calories: 357; Total fat: 25g; Protein: 28g; Sodium: 1,099mg; Fiber: 0g

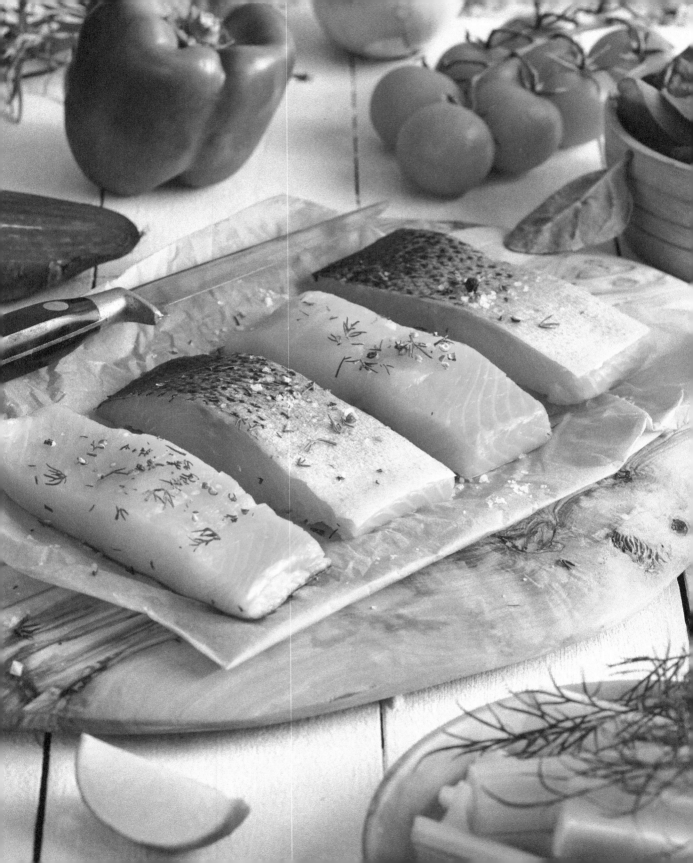

Mini Meatloaf Muffins

Makes 1 dozen muffins   **PREP TIME:** 15 minutes | **COOK TIME:** 20 minutes

These meatloaf muffins freeze well and make a quick and easy complete meal. You can top them with a small amount of shredded cheese prior to baking if you are including dairy in your plan. Leftover muffins are delicious crumbled into marinara sauce (see Easy Marinara Sauce, page 133) and served over zoodles (see the instructions for zucchini noodles in Chicken Thighs with Creamy Arugula Pesto over Zucchini Noodles, page 114) for a heartier meal. You can substitute shredded carrot or parsnip for the zucchini in this recipe, if desired.

1 tablespoon olive oil, for greasing the muffin tin (optional)

1 pound grass-fed ground beef (or organic ground turkey)

1 cup grated/shredded zucchini, all water squeezed out with a paper towel

¼ cup chopped green onion

½ teaspoon garlic powder

1 teaspoon salt

¼ teaspoon freshly ground pepper

2 tablespoons tomato paste (no sugar added)

1 egg, beaten

1. Preheat the oven to 350°F and line a muffin tin with muffin cup liners or coat the cups with olive oil.

2. Place the beef, zucchini, onion, garlic powder, salt, pepper, tomato paste, and egg in a large bowl and combine well with a fork.

3. Place about ¼ cup of the meatloaf mixture into each muffin cup and bake 18 to 20 minutes, until cooked through. Serve warm.

4. Allow the muffins to cool completely before freezing.

PER SERVING (2 Muffins) Calories: 149; Total fat: 8g; Protein: 17g; Sodium: 450mg; Fiber: 0g

Easy Marinara Sauce

Serves 4 to 6   **PREP TIME:** 10 minutes | **COOK TIME:** 35 minutes

It's hard to find a store-bought marinara sauce without added sugar. This is an easy and versatile option to use in many dishes. Serve over zoodles (see the instructions for zucchini noodles in Chicken Thighs with Creamy Arugula Pesto over Zucchini Noodles, page 114) or sautéed green beans or broccoli. Add grilled chicken or ground beef for a heartier meal, if desired. You can double the recipe and freeze half to have on hand.

1 tablespoon olive oil

1 small onion, chopped

1 or 2 carrots, peeled and chopped

2 to 4 garlic cloves, minced

¼ teaspoon salt

Freshly ground black pepper, to taste

32-ounce can crushed tomatoes (with basil, if possible)

2 tablespoons balsamic vinegar

1 teaspoon Italian seasoning

1 cup precooked chicken or ground beef (optional)

2 to 4 tablespoons chopped fresh basil (optional)

1. Heat the oil in a large skillet over medium heat. Add the onion and carrot and sauté until just tender, about 5 minutes.

2. Add the garlic, salt, and pepper, and sauté until fragrant, another 1 to 2 minutes.

3. Reduce the heat to low and add canned tomatoes, balsamic vinegar, Italian seasoning, and chicken or beef (if using). Stir to combine, bring to a simmer, cover, and cook over low heat for 30 minutes to allow the flavors to blend.

4. Add the basil before serving (if using) and serve warm.

PER SERVING Calories: 141; Total fat: 4g; Protein: 6g; Sodium: 595mg; Fiber: 8g

FOOD DIARY: TRACK YOUR REACTIONS

		FOODS	SYMPTOMS
DAY	MORNING		
	AFTERNOON		
	EVENING		
DAY	MORNING		
	AFTERNOON		
	EVENING		
DAY	MORNING		
	AFTERNOON		
	EVENING		

		FOODS	SYMPTOMS
DAY	MORNING		
	AFTERNOON		
	EVENING		
DAY	MORNING		
	AFTERNOON		
	EVENING		
DAY	MORNING		
	AFTERNOON		
	EVENING		

		FOODS	SYMPTOMS
DAY	MORNING		
	AFTERNOON		
	EVENING		
DAY	MORNING		
	AFTERNOON		
	EVENING		
DAY	MORNING		
	AFTERNOON		
	EVENING		

FOODS			SYMPTOMS
DAY	MORNING		
	AFTERNOON		
	EVENING		
DAY	MORNING		
	AFTERNOON		
	EVENING		
DAY	MORNING		
	AFTERNOON		
	EVENING		

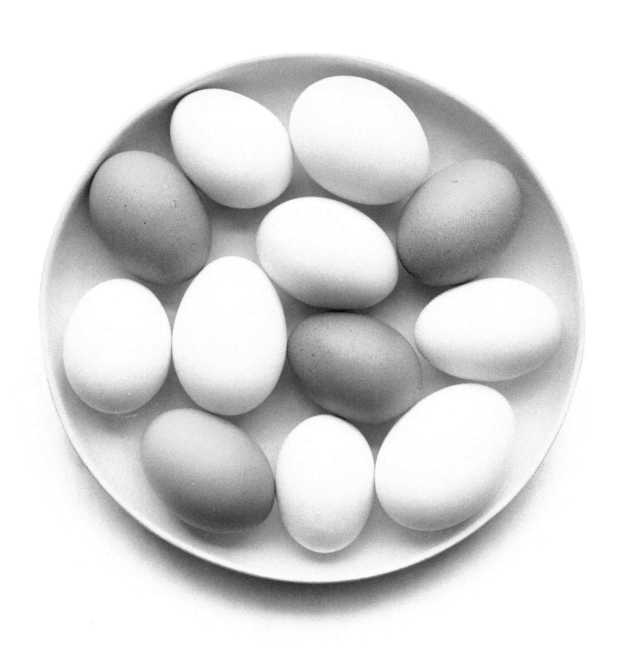

BLANK SHOPPING LIST

VEGETABLES

BEANS / LEGUMES

FRUIT

WHOLE GRAINS

OTHER

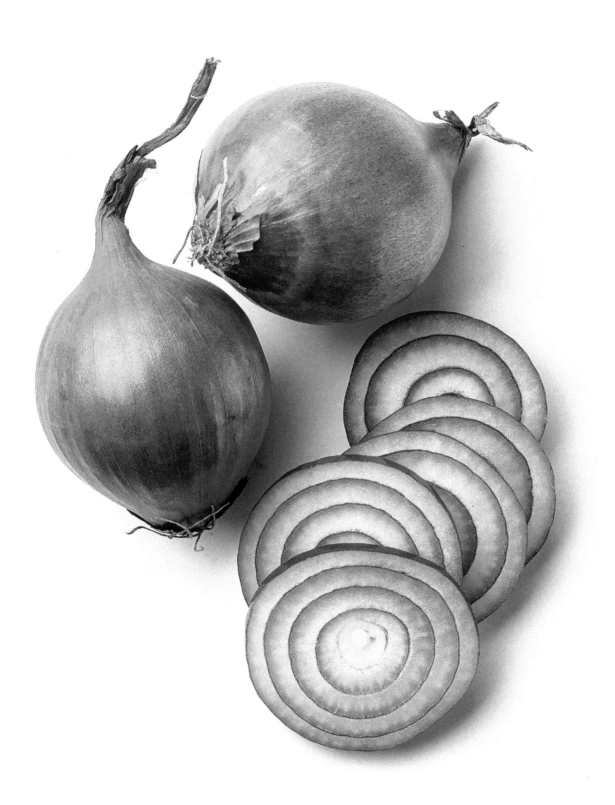

THE DIRTY DOZEN AND THE CLEAN FIFTEEN™

A nonprofit environmental watchdog organization called Environmental Working Group (EWG) looks at data supplied by the US Department of Agriculture (USDA) and the Food and Drug Administration (FDA) about pesticide residues. Each year it compiles a list of the best and worst pesticide loads found in commercial crops. You can use these lists to decide which fruits and vegetables to buy organic to minimize your exposure to pesticides and to see which produce is considered safe enough to buy conventionally. This does not mean they are pesticide-free, though, so wash these fruits and vegetables thoroughly. The list is updated annually, and you can find it online at EWG.org/FoodNews.

Dirty Dozen

1. apples
2. **celery***
3. cherries
4. grapes
5. **kale**
6. **nectarines**
7. peaches
8. pears
9. potatoes
10. **spinach**
11. **strawberries**
12. **tomatoes**

Clean Fifteen

1. **asparagus**
2. **avocados**
3. **broccoli**
4. **cabbages**
5. cantaloupes
6. **cauliflower**
7. sweet corn**
8. **eggplants**
9. kiwis
10. melons, honeydew
11. mushrooms
12. **onions**
13. papayas**
14. sweet peas (frozen)
15. pineapples

---

* **Boldfaced foods** are specifically recommended for the Candida Cleanse.

** A small amount of sweet corn and papaya sold in the United States is produced from genetically modified seeds. Buy organic varieties of these crops if you want to avoid genetically modified produce.

MEASUREMENTS AND CONVERSIONS

VOLUME EQUIVALENTS	US STANDARD	US STANDARD (OUNCES)	METRIC (APPROXIMATE)
LIQUID	2 tablespoons	1 fl. oz.	30 mL
	¼ cup	2 fl. oz.	60 mL
	½ cup	4 fl. oz.	120 mL
	1 cup	8 fl. oz.	240 mL
	1½ cups	12 fl. oz.	355 mL
	2 cups or 1 pint	16 fl. oz.	475 mL
	4 cups or 1 quart	32 fl. oz.	1 L
	1 gallon	128 fl. oz.	4 L
DRY	⅛ teaspoon	–	0.5 mL
	¼ teaspoon	–	1 mL
	½ teaspoon	–	2 mL
	¾ teaspoon	–	4 mL
	1 teaspoon	–	5 mL
	1 tablespoon	–	15 mL
	¼ cup	–	59 mL
	⅓ cup	–	79 mL
	½ cup	–	118 mL
	⅔ cup	–	156 mL
	¾ cup	–	177 mL
	1 cup	–	235 mL
	2 cups or 1 pint	–	475 mL
	3 cups	–	700 mL
	4 cups or 1 quart	–	1 L
	½ gallon	–	2 L
	1 gallon	–	4 L

OVEN TEMPERATURES

FAHRENHEIT	CELSIUS (APPROXIMATE)
250°F	120°C
300°F	150°C
325°F	165°C
350°F	180°C
375°F	190°C
400°F	200°C
425°F	220°C
450°F	230°C

WEIGHT EQUIVALENTS

US STANDARD	METRIC (APPROXIMATE)
½ ounce	15 g
1 ounce	30 g
2 ounces	60 g
4 ounces	115 g
8 ounces	225 g
12 ounces	340 g
16 ounces or 1 pound	455 g

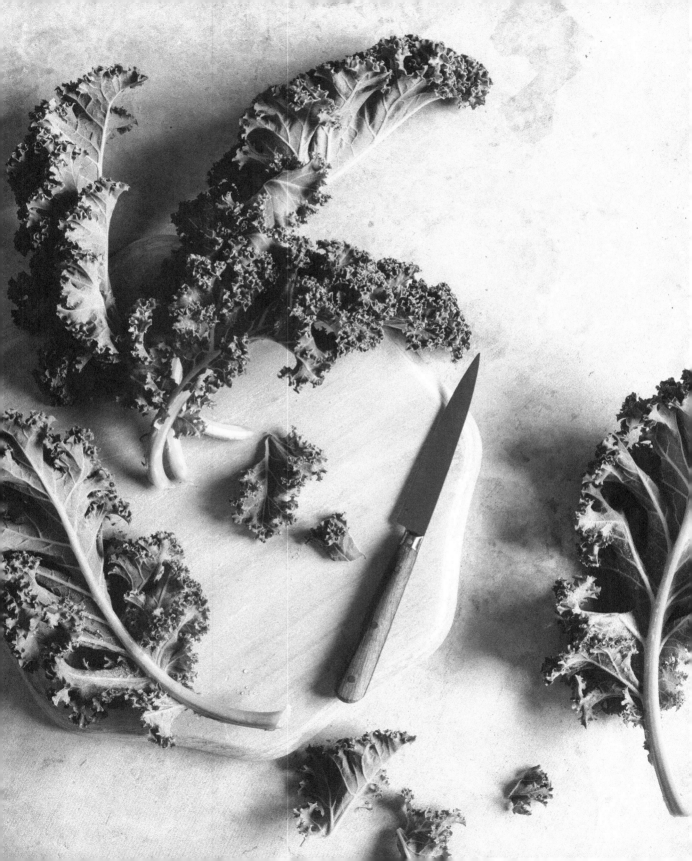

ENDNOTES

1   Knoke, M. and H. Bernhardt. "The First Description of an Oesophageal Candidosis by Bernhard von Langenbeck in 1839." *Mycoses* 49, no. 4 (July 2006): 283-87. doi:10.1111/j.1439-0507.2006.01237.x.

2   Centers for Disease Control and Prevention (CDC). "Candidiasis." Fungal Diseases. N.d. https://www.cdc.gov/fungal/diseases/candidiasis/index.html.

3   Ehrström, Sophia M., Dan Kornfield, Jessica Thuresson, and Eva Rylander. "Signs of Chronic Stress in Women with Recurrent Candida Vulvovaginitis." *American Journal of Obstetrics & Gynecology* 193, no. 4 (Oct. 2005): 1376-1381. doi:10.1016/j.ajog.2005.03.068; Centers for Disease Control and Prevention (CDC). "Medications That Weaken Your Immune System." Fungal Diseases. N.d. https://www.cdc.gov/fungal/infections/immune-system.html; Jabra-Rizk, Mary Ann, Eric F. Kong, Christina Tsui, M. Hong Nguyen, Cornelius J. Clancy, Paul L. Fidel, Jr., Mairi Noverr. "*Candida Albicans* Pathogenesis: Fitting within the Host-Microbe Damage Response Framework.," edited by A. T. Maurelli. *American Society for Microbiology*. Infection and Immunity 84, no. 10 (Sept. 2016): 2724-2739. https://iai.asm.org/content/84/10/2724, doi: 10.1128/IAI.00469-16.

4   Jabra-Rizk, et al. "*Candida Albicans* Pathogenesis."

5   Cleveland Clinic. "Gut-Brain Connection." https://my.clevelandclinic.org/health/treatments/16358-gut-brain-connection.

6   Severance, Emily G., Kristin L. Gressitt, Catherine R. Stallings, Emily Katsafanas, Lucy A. Schweinfurth, Christina L. Savage, Maria B. Adamos, Kevin M. Sweeney, Andrea E. Origoni, Sunil Khushalani, et al. "*Candida alibcans* Exposures, Sex Specificity and Cognitive Deficits in Schizophrenia and Bipolar Disorder." *Nature, NPJ: Schizophrenia* 2 (May 4, 2016): Article no. 16018.

7   Cleveland Clinic. "Gut-Brain Connection." https://my.clevelandclinic.org/health/treatments/16358-gut-brain-connection.

8   Pappas, Peter G., Carol A. Kauffman, David R. Andes, Cornelius J. Clancy, Kieren A. Marr, Luis Ostrosky-Zeichner, Annette C. Reboli, Mindy G. Schuster, Jose A. Vazquez, Thomas J. Walsh, et al. "Clinical Practice Guideline for the Management of Candidiasis: 2016 Update by the Infectious Diseases Society of America." *Clinical Infectious Diseases* 62, no. 4 (Feb. 15, 2016):e1-e50. doi:10.1093/cid/civ933.

9   CDC. "Candidiasis."

[10] Allonsius, Camille N., Marianne F. L. Van den Broek, Ilke De Boeck, Shari Kiekens, Eline F.M. Oerlemans, Filip Kiekens, Kenn Foubert, Dieter Vandenheuvel, Paul Cos, Peter Delputte, et al. "Interplay between *Lactobacillus rhamnosus* GG and *Candida* and the Involvement of Exopolysaccharides." *Microbial Biotechnology* 10, no. 6 (2017): 1753-63. doi:10.1111/1751-7915.12799; Murina, Filippo, Alessandra Graziottin, Francesco De Seta. "Can *Lactobacillus fermentum* LF10 and *Lactobacillus acidophilus* LA02 in a Slow-Release Vaginal Product Be Useful for Prevention of Recurrent Vulvovaginal Candidiasis?: A Clinical Study. *Journal of Clinical Gastroenterology* 48, supp. 1 (Nov.–Dec. 2014): S102-05. doi:10.1097/MCG.0000000000000225; Kumar, Suresh, Arun Bansal, and Sunit Singhi. "Evaluation of Efficacy of Probiotics in Prevention of Candida Colonization in a PICU-a Randomized Controlled Trial." *Critical Care Medicine* 41, no. 2 (Feb. 2013): 565-72. doi:10.1097/CCM.0b013e31826a409c; Santos, Agda Lima dos, Jorge Antônio Olavo Cardoso, Silvana Soléo Ferreira dos Santos, Silva Célia Regina Gonçalves, and Leão Mariella Vieira Pereira. "Influence of Probiotics on *Candida* Presence and IgA Anti-*Candida* in the Oral Cavity." *Brazilian Journal of Microbiology* 40, no. 4 (2009): 960-64. doi:10.1590/S1517-83822009000400030; Chew, S. Y., Y. K. Cheah, H. F. Seow, Doblin Sandai, and L. Than. "Probiotic *Lactobacillus rhamnosus* GR-1 and *Lactobacillus reuteri* RC-14 Exhibit Strong Antifungal Effects Against Vulvovaginal Candidiasis-Causing *Candida glabrata* Isolates." *Journal of Applied Microbiology* 118, no. 5 (May 2015): 1180-90. doi:10.1111/jam.12772.

[11] Allonsius et al. "Interplay between *Lactobacillus rhamnosus* GG and *Candida*"; Murina et al. "Can *Lactobacillus fermentum* LF10 and *Lactobacillus acidophilus* LA02"; Kumar et al. "Evaluation of Efficacy of Probiotics"; Santos et al. "Influence of Probiotics on *Candida* Presence"; Chew et al. "Probiotic *Lactobacillus rhamnosus* GR-1 and *Lactobacillus reuteri* RC-14."

[12] Webb, Denise. "Phytochemicals' Role in Good Health." *Today's Dietitian* 15, no. 9 (Sept. 2013): 70. https://www.todaysdietitian.com/newarchives/090313p70.shtml.

[13] Jacob, Aglaée. "Treatment and Management of SIBO—Taking a Dietary Approach Can Control Intestinal Fermentation and Inflammation." *Today's Dietitian* 14, no. 12 (Dec. 2012): 16. https://www.todaysdietitian.com/newarchives/121112p16.shtml.

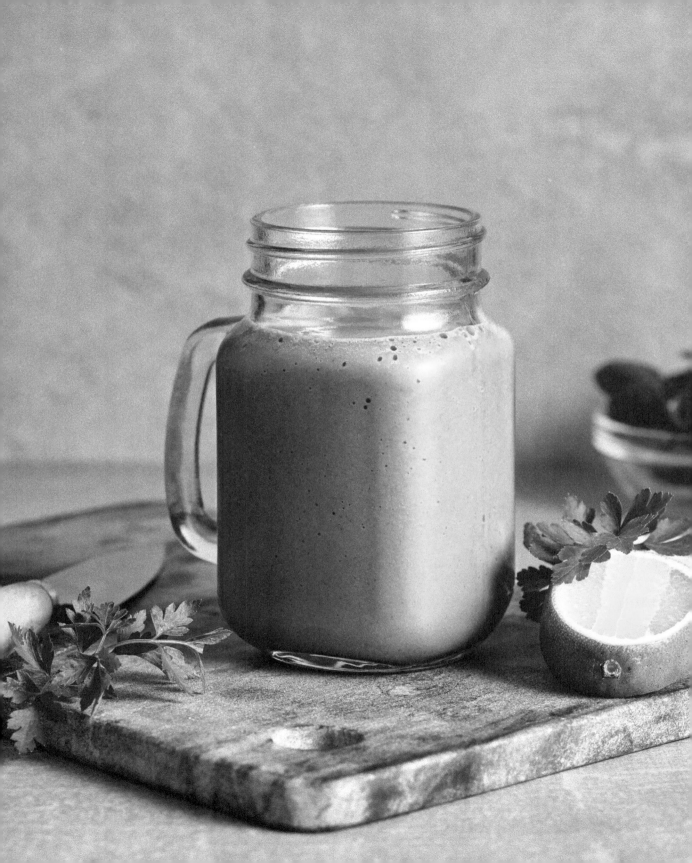

RECIPE INDEX

INDEX

ACKNOWLEDGMENTS

A heartfelt thank you to all the beautiful patients I have had the privilege of working with across my career. You are the reason I love what I do every day and continuously strive to learn more, uncover new answers, and test developing theories. I am so grateful for the trust you have put in me and my approach and the efforts you have made to walk the path toward better health. Each and every one of you are strong and hold a place in my heart.

To my family: my rock. I have parents who have endlessly supported me through every journey I have taken that has led me to this point in my career. I cannot thank you enough for being loving role models of empathy and determination. I have an admirably patient husband who has offered me encouragement through every step of the way; I am a stronger person with you in my life. And Harper, Luke, and Evan, I am so grateful for your adventurous palates that have allowed me to always be creative in the kitchen. I also appreciate your brutal honesty!

To the pioneers in integrative and functional medicine who looked beyond traditional therapies to explore the root cause of illness and focus on healing the whole person, inside and out. You have provided inspiration, experience, and so much knowledge to my practice.

I am grateful for my editor, Marisa Hines, and her fantastic team at Callisto Media who have made all the little details come alive, allowing me to focus on what I do best: healing through nutrition.

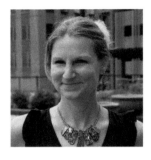 **Molly Devine** is a registered dietitian who specializes in digestive health, healthy weight management, and chronic disease prevention through integrative and functional nutrition. She is an advocate for sustainable lifestyle change through nutrition intervention and the founder of Eat Your Keto, a nutrition counseling and individualized meal planning service focusing on therapeutic whole foods-based diets for disease prevention and management. She is the co-author of *The Ketogenic Lifestyle: How to Fuel Your Best* and a regular contributor to nutrition-based online media such as *Shape* magazine, *Insider, Greatist, The Huffington Post, Brides* magazine, and ABC11 Eyewitness News.

Molly received her bachelor's degree in nutrition sciences from North Carolina Central University and completed her dietetic internship through Meredith College. She also holds a bachelor's degree in languages and linguistics from Georgetown University. She lives in Durham, North Carolina, with her family.